INTRODUCTION TO HUMAN IMMUNOLOGY

TERESA L. HUFFER, R.N.
Shady Grove Adventist Hospital, Gaithersburg, Maryland, and
Frederick Community College, Frederick, Maryland

DOROTHY J. KANAPA, M.B.A.
National Cancer Institute, Frederick, Maryland

GEORGE W. STEVENSON, M.D.
Northwestern University Medical Center, Chicago, Illinois

JONES AND BARTLETT PUBLISHERS, INC.
Boston Portola Valley

Editorial offices: Jones and Bartlett Publishers, Inc., 30 Granada Court, Portola Valley, CA 94025.
Sales and customer service offices: Jones and Bartlett Publishers, Inc., 20 Park Plaza, Boston, MA 02116.

Library of Congress Cataloging in Publication Data

Huffer, Teresa L.
Introduction to human immunology.

Includes bibliographies and index.
1. Immunology. 2. Immunologic diseases.
I. Kanapa, Dorothy J. II. Stevenson, George W.
III. Title. [DNLM: 1. Immune System. 2. Immunologic Diseases. QW 504 H899i]
QR181.H79 1986 616.07'9 86-2849

ISBN 0-86720-067-7 (pbk.)

STAFF FOR THIS BOOK
Consulting editor: Henry C. Stevenson, M.D.
Copy editor: Leesa M. Stanion
Production and design: Elizabeth W. Thomson
Illustrations: Deborah Schneck
Cover design: D.J. Kanapa

PREFACE

Immunology is a century-old science that attempts to define and characterize the organ system responsible for protecting the human body from invasion by nonself (foreign) organisms such as bacteria, fungi, and viruses, or altered-self cell types such as tumor cells. Clinical applications of immunology have developed at many different levels over the last 50 years, ranging from immunotherapy for allergic diseases to the treatment of catastrophic immunologic-related diseases (diseases that affect the immune system) such as rheumatoid arthritis and systemic lupus erythematosis. The advent of transplantation surgery in the 1970s brought with it the need for a better understanding of the human immune system and how to manipulate its function to increase acceptance of organ grafts. Radically new therapeutic modalities for cancer and other related diseases were introduced in the 1980s. These treatments manipulate a patient's immune system by the infusion of substances such as interferon, interleukin 2, LAK cells, and monoclonal antibodies. In addition, several new diseases that have emerged over the last 10 years represent catastrophic aberrations of normal human immune functions (for example, acquired immunodeficiency syndrome (AIDS), Lyme arthritis, and eosinophilic fascitis). The nature of these diseases is a source of increasing public concern which, in turn, is becoming a catalyst for the introduction of basic immunologic concepts in the clinical setting.

The high technology currently associated with clinical applications of basic human immunology can be very confusing to professionals and lay persons alike. Recent interest in the science of immunology has created a strong need among individuals of widely diverse backgrounds for comprehensible and up-to-date information about the function of the immune system. These people include individuals at the doctoral level without immunology training, nursing personnel and other allied health professionals, laboratory technicians, and the ever increasing number of business experts who require detailed information about this constantly evolving science.

Our major goal in designing this text is to impart the basic concepts of the science of immunology rapidly and in a manner that is understandable to all students regardless of their backgrounds. This is a Zero Information Based (ZIB™) text. ZIB™ means that we do not assume the reader has any specific background in the sciences. Each scientific term is defined as it is introduced. The reader with some science background at any particular level may just skim the material until an area of new material is encountered. Self-testing questions are provided at the end of each chapter, and we hope that readers will perceive this material as a self-instructional manual.

A second goal of this manual is to clarify the language of immunology, so that the reader may become conversant with immunologists at the doctoral level. We hope to build the reader's confidence to pursue further reading and learning in the field of immunology by tearing down the scientific language barrier that often separates the novice from the expert. Each basic concept is represented by carefully selected figures. We hope this extensive pictorial imagery will encourage readers to visualize and finally to verbalize each concept presented in the text. Our experience has been that students who focus carefully on the figures, verbalize out loud the answers to the questions at the end of each chapter, and learn each concept with the intention of teaching it to others will glean the most from this text. For more detailed technical reading in the field of immunology, supplemental reading lists are provided at the end of each chapter.

Our final goal in preparing this text is to provide a basic understanding of the major immunologic diseases and their treatments (Chapters 25–28). Although a text of this size cannot be comprehensive, a great deal of the latest information in the field is presented. We hope that readers beginning with the basic science chapters will bear in mind that an overview of the impact of immunology at the human level is provided in the final chapters. Our experience with students has been that this perspective vastly enhances the relevance of the information presented here for clinicians and nonclinicians alike.

T.L. Huffer
D.J. Kanapa
G.W. Stevenson

We gratefully acknowledge helpful comments from the following reviewers of the manuscript for this book: Robert I. Mishell, M.D., University of California at Berkeley; Henry R. Hilgard, M.D., University of California at Santa Cruz; Mary Wise, North Virginia Community College, Alexandria; Jack P. Kildebeck, Bakersfield College; Robert J. Egan, Golden West College; Peter Gauthier, Mount Saint Mary's College; Sam W. Joseph, University of Maryland; Don Steinert, Robert D. Young, and Margaret R. Peterson, R.N., Columbia Union College; Agnes A. Kemerer, R.N., Frederick Community College; Linda L. Blackwood, San Francisco State University; Gabriel Virella, M.D., Medical University of South Carolina; William D. Stansfield, California Polytechnical State University; Ann Baldwin, Richard Davey, M.D., and Linda Muul, National Institutes of Health; N. D. Gary and S. J. Silverman, Hood College; Sandra Bronson, National Institute of Allergy and Infectious Diseases.

CONTENTS

DEDICATION

To Teresa, Jo Ann, Paul, Margie, Audrey, Cindy, Steve, Leo, and our many other friends who helped close the language barrier and open channels of communication in our bioscience research group. In addition, we are eternally indebted to the most powerful teaching forces in our lives—our parents.

PART I

BIOCHEMISTRY OF THE IMMUNE SYSTEM

The human body is made up of various cooperating cellular units called **organs**. Organs maintain an environment conducive to the life of all the body's cells. The master organ of the body is the brain, where consciousness exists and without which human life cannot exist. All of the other organ systems are support mechanisms to keep the environment of the body normal so that the brain can function optimally. In this book, we are going to study the **immune system**, one particular support system responsible for protecting the body, or "self," from invasion by "nonself"—bacteria, viruses, cancer cells, or other foreign matter.

The immune system, like all other systems in the body, is composed of distinct types of cells. In this chapter, we present the basic chemistry required for an understanding of how the building blocks of cells (biomolecules) are assembled and how they interact to form a living cell. Because antibodies, antigens, interferon, and the many other components of the immune system are relatively complicated biomolecules, it is important to feel secure about basic chemistry and biochemistry before proceeding. After mastering this material, you will be prepared to learn the details of the anatomy and function of the immune system. Please remember, do not focus only on the concepts; it is also very important to verbalize out loud the scientific terminology (language).

CHAPTER 1

ATOMIC THEORY

All cells and the biomolecules of which cells are made are composed of basic particles known as **atoms**. Atoms are the building blocks of all matter and are composed of three fundamental subatomic particles: **electrons**, **protons**, and **neutrons**, as seen in Figure 1–1. These three subatomic particles can be distinguished on the basis of their weight and their electrical charge. The proton has a positive charge, the electron has a negative charge, and the neutron has no charge. Positive charges attract negative charges (and vice versa), but positive charges repel other positive charges and negative charges repel other negative charges. The electrons can be visualized as moving around the outside of the **nucleus** (the central core of the atom) in a pattern known as an orbit (Figure 1–1). Electrons are attracted to protons, which are inside the nucleus. Although the speed of the electrons in the orbit tends to propel the electrons away from the nucleus, the electrical attraction between the protons and the electrons holds the electrons in a stable orbit. In atoms that have more than one proton (most atoms), the forces that hold the protons together in the nucleus are not entirely known. These forces are called strong nuclear forces or **quarks**. The attraction between the protons, which are located in the nucleus, and the electrons, which are moving in their orbits, is the major force holding atoms together. When two different atomic nuclei with positively charged protons have an attraction for the *same set* of electrons, a **molecular bond** (linkage) is formed between the two atoms. Understanding molecular bonds is essential to understanding biochemistry because **molecules**, which are atoms linked together by chemical bonds, are the building blocks for all types of cells and biological materials.

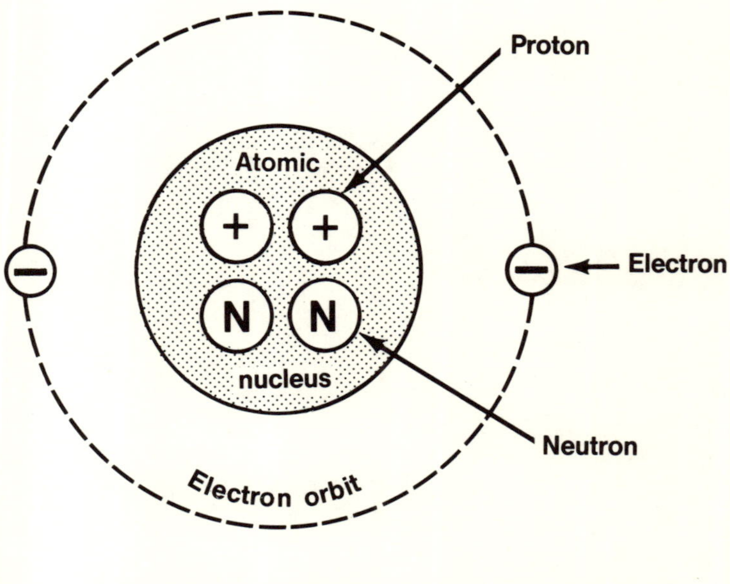

Figure 1–1. Organization of subatomic particles in an atom.

Subatomic particles—protons, neutrons, and electrons—differ not only in charge but also in weight. In order to understand the concept of weight regarding atomic matter, you must understand the concept of a **mole**. One mole equals a specific number of particles; the specific number is 602,000,000,000,000,000,000,000 or 6.02 x 10^{23} in scientific notation. Instead of referring to this cumbersome number numerically, we simply use the term "one mole" (just as one dozen is equal to 12 items). Neutrons and protons weigh the same; specifically, one mole of protons or one mole of neutrons weighs one gram. In contrast, electrons weigh very little: one mole of electrons weighs about one two-thousandth of a gram.

In summary, atoms are composed of three types of subatomic particles: positively charged protons, neutrons that have no charge, and negatively charged electrons. Protons and neutrons are found in the center of the nucleus of the atom, and the electrons orbit around the nucleus. These concepts are summarized in Table 1–1.

Table 1–1. Characteristics of Subatomic Particles.

Particle Type	Charge	Location in Atom	Weight
Proton	Positive	Nucleus	1 gram/mole
Neutron	Neutral	Nucleus	1 gram/mole
Electron	Negative	Orbiting nucleus	No significant weight

The atom with its nucleus and orbiting electrons is the basic unit of all matter. There are 106 known types of atoms, and each type represents one of the 106 basic types of material known to exist on the earth. The 106 atoms or materials are called **elements**. The lightest element (of least atomic weight) is hydrogen; an atom of hydrogen has only 1 proton in its nucleus. An atom of the heaviest element has 106 protons in its nucleus. *The characteristics of each element are directly related to the number of protons in the nucleus of the atoms of that element.* It is impossible to change the number of protons in the nucleus of an atom of an element without changing the element completely; thus, if one proton is added to the nucleus of hydrogen (which contains only one proton) the hydrogen atom is automatically transformed into an atom of a new element—helium.

The number of neutrons, as opposed to protons, in the nucleus of each atom is not predictable. A change in the number of neutrons in the nucleus of each atom does not affect the overall reaction characteristics of the atom, *except* that when too many neutrons are added the atom can become radioactive. These atoms are called **radioactive isotopes**.

From a biochemical perspective, the most important subatomic particles are the *electrons*. These particles have negligible weight in comparison to the protons and neutrons, and they have a negative charge. Because they move so fast around the nucleus, there is a tendency for them to escape the nucleus. However, the attraction of the electrons to the positively charged protons works to counteract this tendency and to hold them in an orbit around the nucleus. The attraction by protons from two different atomic nuclei for the *same set* of electrons is the basis for the **bonds** that hold molecules together.

Try to visualize the atom as a unit composed of three types of subatomic particles: neutrons and protons in a nucleus, with electrons orbiting outside. Because the weight of the protons and the neutrons is known (one gram per one mole of each subatomic particle) and because the weight of the electrons is negligible, it then becomes very easy to calculate the weight of one mole of any type of atom. To do this, simply determine the number of protons (one gram per mole for each proton) and the number of neutrons (one gram per mole for each neutron) in the nucleus of that atom. The sum of the numbers of protons and neutrons multiplied by one gram per mole equals the **atomic weight**. For example, helium has two protons and two neutrons. Therefore, the atomic weight is $(2 + 2) \times$ 1 gram per mole = an atomic weight of 4 grams per mole. Because electrons weigh so little, they generally do not enter into the calculation of atomic weight.

The 106 elements are arranged in a particular order based on the number of protons in the nucleus of each atom of each element. The **atomic number** is the number of protons in the nucleus of each atom of the element. Thus, hydrogen (atomic number 1) has one proton in its nucleus, helium (atomic number 2) has two protons in its nucleus, and so forth. Figure 1–2 is an abbreviated periodic table containing the first 18 known elements. These elements are ordered according to their atomic number, which reflects the number of protons in the nucleus of each atom. Remember that the number of protons in the nucleus of an atom cannot be changed without changing that atom to a completely different type of atom. Under the atomic number, you will find the name of the element, and in parentheses you will find the abbreviation used to represent the element. Finally, at the bottom of each box, you will find the atomic weight, that is, the weight in grams per mole of one mole of that atom, derived by multiplying the number of protons and neutrons in the nucleus of that atom by one gram per mole. When you know the atomic number of an atom, you automatically know the number of protons in that atom and can therefore calculate the number of neutrons in the nucleus: simply subtract the number of protons in the atom (the atomic number) from the total atomic weight; the remaining number is the number of neutrons in the nucleus of each atom of that element. This information will be utilized in the next chapter to understand the bonding characteristics of atoms and the overall weight of atoms bonded together (to form molecules).

Suggested Reading

Ouellette, R. J. *Introduction to General, Organic and Biological Chemistry*. New York: Macmillan, 1984.

Widom, J. M. and S. J. Edelstein. *Chemistry*. San Francisco: Freeman, 1981.

REVIEW QUESTIONS for Atomic Theory

1. What are atoms?

Atoms are the building blocks of matter. Pure forms of a type of atom (like pure gold, iron, mercury) are known as elements. [p. 2]

2. How many types of elements are currently known?

There are 106 elements currently known. [p. 3]

3. Describe the three basic components of an atom and their relative positions.

The three basic components of atoms are electrons, protons, and neutrons. The protons and neutrons cluster together at the center of the atom to form an atomic nucleus. The electrons move around the nucleus in patterns known as orbits. [p. 2]

I	II	III	IV	V	VI	VII	VIII
Atomic number = 1 Hydrogen [H] Atomic weight = [1]							2 Helium [He] [4]
3 Lithium [Li] [7]	4 Beryllium [Be] [9]	5 Boron [B] [11]	6 Carbon [C] [12]	7 Nitrogen [N] [14]	8 Oxygen [O] [16]	9 Fluorine [F] [19]	10 Neon [N] [20]
11 Sodium [Na] [23]	12 Magnesium [Mg] [24]	13 Aluminum [Al] [27]	14 Silicon [Si] [28]	15 Phosphorus [P] [31]	16 Sulfur [S] [32]	17 Chlorine [Cl] [35]	18 Argon [Ar] [40]
Elements 19–106 are not shown in this table.							

Figure 1–2. Abbreviated periodic table of the elements.

4. What is the major difference between electrons, protons, and neutrons? Explain.

One major difference among all three is their respective electrical charges. The electron has a negative electrical charge, the proton has a positive charge, and the neutron is neutral, having no charge. In addition, protons and neutrons weigh the same (1 gram per mole); electrons have negligible weight. [p. 3]

5. What is the major effect of an electrical charge?

The major effect is to exert a force upon other electrical charges in the vicinity. There is an attractive force between charges of an opposite nature, i.e., a positive and a negative charge attract one another, while there is a repulsive force between charges of a similar nature, i.e., two positive or two negative charges will repel each other. [p. 3]

6. What are molecules?

Molecules are individual atoms linked together by chemical bonds (a shared set of electrons). [p. 2]

7. What is a mole?

A mole is a fixed number of a type of particle (such as atoms or molecules). The specific number is 602,000,000,000,000,000,000,000 (6.02×10^{23} in scientific notation). [p. 3]

8. What is the atomic number?

The atomic number is the number of protons that a particular atom has in its nucleus. [p. 4]

9. What is the atomic weight?

The atomic weight is a measure of the weight of an atom. A mole of protons weighs 1 gram; neutrons also weigh 1 gram per mole. A mole of electrons weighs almost nothing. The weight of a mole of any type of atom simply reflects the number of protons and neutrons in a mole of that atom. Thus, 1 mole of hydrogen = 1 mole of protons = 1 gram per mole = atomic weight, and 1 mole of carbon = 6 moles of protons + 6 moles of neutrons = 12 grams per mole = atomic weight. [p. 3]

CHAPTER 2

ELECTRONS AND THEIR ORBITS

We now turn our attention to the most important subatomic particle in the atom, the *electron*. **Chemistry** is the study of the electrons orbiting the nucleus and how the electrons of each atom interact to form chemical bonds; so it stands to reason that electrons are the focus of chemistry. The characteristics of electron bonding tendencies of each element are the reason that the periodic table is arranged in column form, with the elements in each column, I through VIII, all demonstrating the same type of electron reactivity pattern (ability to form bonds).

To understand atomic electron reactivity, a few background concepts are needed. First, atoms in their baseline state have no overall charge; they have the same number of electrons as protons, and because the positive and negative charges balance each other, the overall charge of the total atom is neutral. Thus, to calculate the number of electrons that a stable atom possesses, simply remember that the neutral atom contains the same number of electrons as it does protons (the atomic number). Electrons can be visualized as moving around the nucleus in spherical orbits known as **shells**. Each shell represents a certain energy level. As shown in Figure 2–1, the lowest energy shell, called the *K shell*, can contain only two electrons; if an atom possesses more than two electrons, the first two electrons must be placed in the K shell and the remaining electrons in the

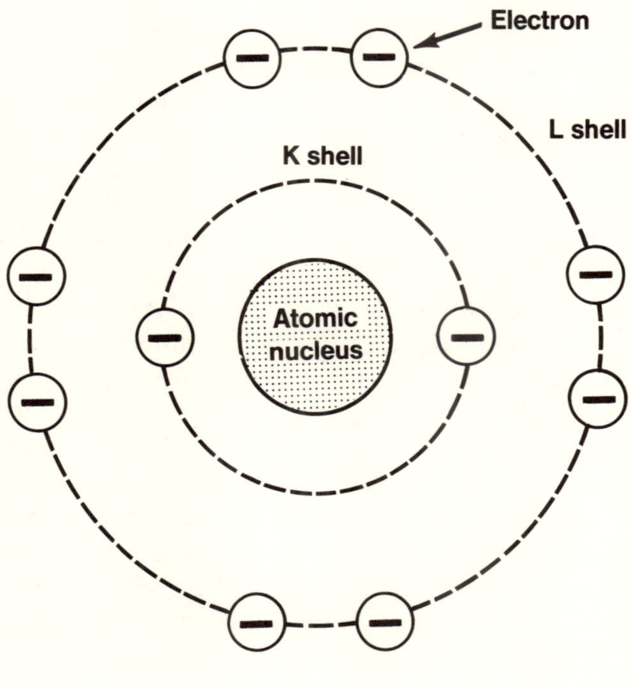

Figure 1–2. Abbreviated periodic table of the elements.

next energy level—the *L shell.* The L shell can hold a maximum of eight electrons before it becomes filled. (We will not discuss any other electron energy shells because the bioelements that we will discuss have fewer than 10 electrons.)

To determine a particular element's **electron configuration**, you take its atomic number, which equals the number of protons in the nucleus and also equals the number of electrons in the neutral atom, and place the appropriate number of electrons in the appropriate shells. All of the electrons in each shell stay a maximal distance apart from one another because they repel one another.

To help understand the periodic table, the most important column to remember is column VIII. The atoms in this column are the **inert gases**—helium, neon and argon, for example. These unusual, stable elements are considered inert because they will not react (form bonds) with any other atom to form molecules. They will not share electrons, give up electrons, or lose electrons to any other atom because their outer valence shells are completely filled. This is important because all of the other elements on the periodic table would like to mimic the stability (filled outer valence shells) of the nearest inert gas element. For example, the element fluorine, which is one electron away from looking like neon, would like to *gain* just one more electron in some manner in order to have a completed L shell and thus be able to mimic neon. Similarly, the element lithium has one electron in the L shell; it would like to *lose* that electron so that it would have a completed K shell just like helium. If you look closely at all of the elements in the periodic table, you can see that all of the elements in each column have the same tendencies with regard to gaining or losing electrons. All the elements in column VII would like to *gain* one electron to look like the nearest inert gas, and all of the elements in column I would like to *lose* one electron to look like the nearest inert gas. Similarly, all of the elements in column VI would like to gain two electrons to look like the nearest inert gas, and so on.

An atom that gains or loses an electron is called an **ion**. If an atom gains one electron, it assumes an additional negative charge and is represented by its atomic symbol with a minus sign. All negatively charged ions are called **anions**. As shown in Figure 2–2, for example, fluorine (atomic number = 9) ordinarily has nine electrons orbiting the nucleus (electrons are numbered 1 to 9). When an additional electron is added to the L shell, the atom has a *net negative* charge (more electrons than protons) and becomes the fluoride ion, abbreviated F^-. If an atom loses an electron, it lacks one electrical charge and the atom has a *net positive* charge and is represented by its atomic symbol with a plus sign. For example, lithium, with an atomic number of 3, ordinarily has three electrons; #1 and #2 are in the K shell, and #3 is in the L shell. When one electron is removed (#3), the L shell becomes empty and the atom becomes the lithium ion (abbreviated Li^+). All positively charged ions are called **cations**.

How many electrons are available in the outer *valence* shell for bonding (or sharing between two atoms), and where these electrons are located (the sites of future bonds), are concerns of great importance when considering the electron structure of each atom. To demonstrate this, let us now focus on the **four principal bioelements**—**hydrogen** (H), **carbon** (C), **nitrogen** (N), and **oxygen** (O). These are the most important atoms to understand because they constitute over 95 percent of all the atoms found in the molecules of the human body. These four bioelements are the building blocks of all biomolecules. We ask that you remember the details of these four elements, shown in Table 2–1, in order to understand the chemical reactions involving these elements.

Hydrogen is the first bioelement to consider. Hydrogen has one proton in its nucleus, as shown in Figure 2–3. A single electron orbits in the shell nearest the nucleus—the K shell. Hydrogen would like either to gain one more electron in order to mimic the nearest inert gas, helium, or to lose one electron and not have any electrons whatsoever (also a stable state).

The next bioelement to consider is *carbon*. Carbon has six protons and six neutrons in its nucleus, and six electrons orbiting the nucleus. In Figure 2–3, electrons #1 and #2 are placed in the inner K shell, opposite one another because

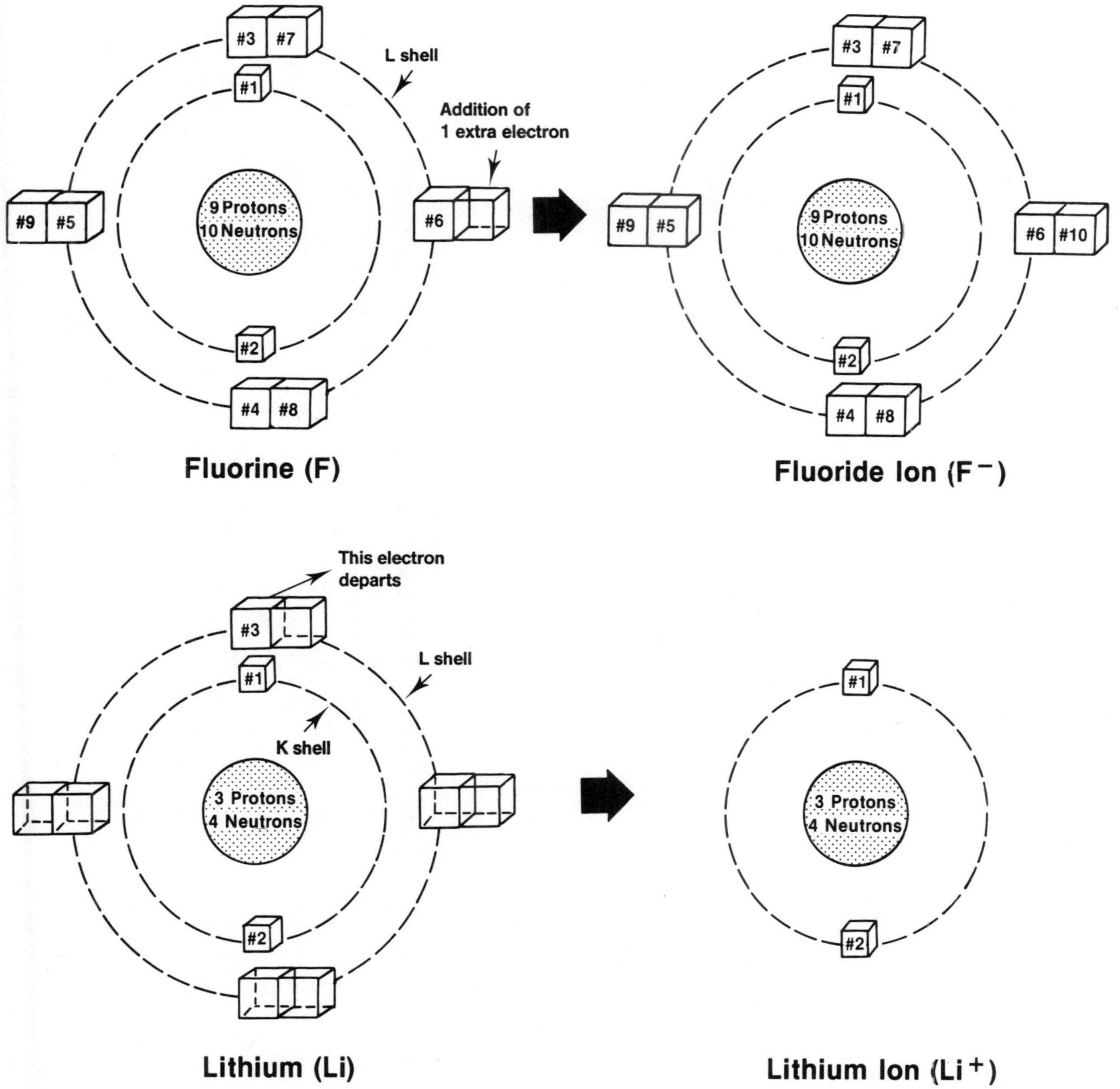

Figure 2–2. Formation of the fluoride anion and the lithium cation.

Table 2–1. Characteristics of the Four Bioelements.

Bioelement	*Symbol*	*Atomic Number*	*Total Number of Protons*	*Total Number of Electrons*	*Valence Electrons Available for Binding*
Hydrogen	**H**	**1**	**1**	**1**	**1**
Carbon	**C**	**6**	**6**	**6**	**4**
Nitrogen	**N**	**7**	**7**	**7**	**3**
Oxygen	**O**	**8**	**8**	**8**	**2**

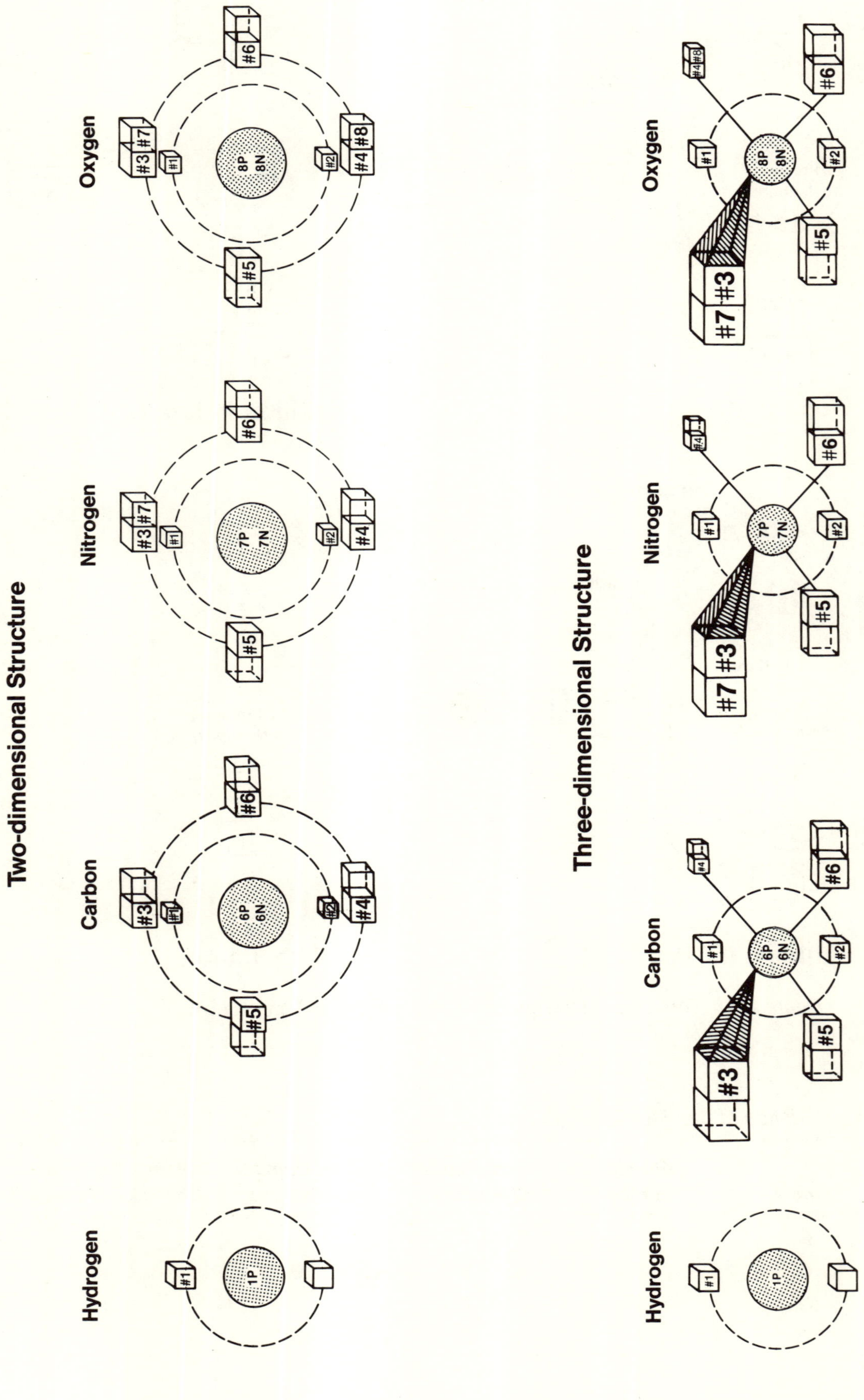

Figure 2–3. The two-dimensional and three-dimensional structure of the bioelements.

of their mutual repulsion. The other four electrons (#3, #4, #5, and #6) are placed in the L shell. Note the arrangement of these electrons: #3 is at the top of the outer shell, #4 is at the bottom, #5 is on the left side, and #6 is on the right side of the shell. Carbon needs to gain four more electrons in order to have the same stable manner of electrons (eight) as neon. Alternatively, it could lose four electrons and mimic helium with two electrons in the K shell. However, carbon is an extremely stable atom—it does not want either to gain or to lose electrons. Please note that the electrons in the L shell are grouped *in four pair group spaces*. Only after all of the four pair group spaces have one electron can the second electron to each group space then be added, until the entire L shell is filled. The four electron pairs repel one another as if they were single electrons; there is no simple explanation for why the two electrons in a pair group do not repel one another. Carbon has four single, unpaired electrons in its outer shell. In Figure 2–3, note the empty squares; these are spaces that may be occupied by the electrical interaction of electrons from another atom, forming shared electron pairs called chemical or **electron bonds**.

The third bioelement to consider is *nitrogen*. Nitrogen has seven protons and seven neutrons in its nucleus. Note that nitrogen also has seven electrons: #1 and #2 are in the inner K shell; #3, #4, #5, and #6 are equally spaced around the outer L shell. As seen in Figure 2–3, nitrogen's seventh electron is placed next to the third electron, in the topmost electron pair space. Thus, nitrogen has only three unpaired electrons in its outer shell and would like to gain three more electrons to be like the nearest inert gas, neon. Because nitrogen has only three unpaired electrons in its outer shell, it is capable of forming only three bonds with other atoms.

Finally, consider the bioelement *oxygen*. It has eight protons and eight neutrons in its nucleus, and eight orbiting electrons. Electrons #1 and #2 are in the inner K shell; #3, #4, #5, #6, #7, and #8 are placed in the L shell. Note in Figure 2–3 that electron #7 is placed beside electron #3, and electron #8 alongside electron #4. This leaves only two electron spaces with a single unpaired electron, spaces which are located to the right and left of the nucleus. Thus, oxygen needs to gain only two electrons to mimic the nearest inert gas, neon, and is capable of forming only two chemical bonds.

The two-dimensional representations of the orientations of electrons around the nucleus in space are idealized. Although the four electron pair spaces appear to be maximally distant from one another in two dimensions, it turns out that in three dimensions they are not. Unfortunately, it is difficult to describe verbally the exact orientation of the four electron pair spaces around the atoms of carbon, nitrogen, and oxygen in the L electron shell. A pictorial description is provided as a model (Figure 2–4) of a carbon atom that can be folded to show the three-dimensional orientation of the bonding electrons around the carbon nucleus. Once assembled, tilt the top of the pyramidal structure toward you so that the #3 electron group is closer to you than the #5 and #6 electron groups; the #4 electron group faces directly away from you. The three-dimensional model represents the approximate orientation of the electron groups in space. The electron groups are not separated from one another by 90° angles (as in the two-dimensional model) but by angles that are closer to 110°. This orientation of the 4 electron groups in space around the carbon nucleus is called a **tetrahedral arrangement** and represents the maximal possible separation of electron groups. Returning to Figure 2–3, you will find the two-dimensional electron structure of hydrogen, carbon, nitrogen, and oxygen, and our pictorial representation of their three-dimensional structures as well. In contrast to the two-dimensional representation where the electron pairs are each at 90° to one another with reference to the nucleus, in the three-dimensional form, the electron pairs are *actually* closer to 110° from one another. This arrangement is known as a **tetrahedral structure**. We have represented this three-dimensionally by showing two of the electron pairs in the same dimension as the paper itself; lines going from the nucleus to the electron pair form an inverted V. The other two electron pairs form a V shape at the top of the nucleus. However, as is evident in the model, one of the electron pairs comes out toward the viewer (as shown in Figure 2–3 by the large line and large electron numbers), and another electron pair goes back behind the sheet of paper (as shown by the small line and small electron numbers). Thus, in a three-dimensional tetrahedral configuration, all of the electron pairs are approximately 110° from one another; this is the maximum distance that the electron pairs can repel one another in space.

In summary, hydrogen has one electron located in its K shell, which is available for bonding (forming an electron pair). Carbon has four electrons available for bonding. Each electron occupies one of the four electron pair spaces located in a tetrahedral arrangement around the carbon nucleus; because each electron is unpaired, there is a possibility of forming four bonds with other atoms. Nitrogen has five electrons in its outer shell; one of the electron pair spaces is filled with two electrons, and thus no bond can form there. However, the three other electron pair spaces have a single unpaired electron in each of them, available for bonding. The three unpaired electrons are located in a pyramidal arrangement to one side of the nucleus of nitrogen; the electron pair space on the other side of the nucleus is filled. Oxygen has six electrons in its outer shell; two of the four electron pair spaces are filled, and thus only two unpaired electrons are available for bonding. The unpaired electrons are arranged in an inverted V configuration with the nucleus—they are not in a straight line. The electron pair sites around carbon, nitrogen, and oxygen are in a tetrahedral arrangement; in oxygen, two of those four electron pair sites are filled, leaving only two unpaired electrons, arranged in an inverted V.

Suggested Reading

Ouellette, R. J. *Introduction to General, Organic and Biological Chemistry*. New York: Macmillan, 1984.

Widom, J. M. and S. J. Edelstein. *Chemistry*. San Francisco: Freeman, 1981.

REVIEW QUESTIONS for Electrons and Their Orbits

1. What is chemistry?

Chemistry is the study of electrons around an atom and how they form bonds between atoms. [p. 7]

2. What is the electrical charge of an atom?

The atom as a whole is electrically neutral because for every positive proton that an atom contains there is one negative electron. Neutrons have no charge. [p. 7]

3. How are electrons placed around an atom?

In orbits called shells, each shell representing a different energy level. [p. 7]

4. Will elements in column I of the periodic chart tend to gain or lose electrons? How many? Why? What type of ion will they become?

Elements in column I will tend to lose one electron. It will be easier to lose the one electron in the outside (valence) shell, allowing them to have the same number of electrons in the outer shell as does the nearest inert gas. They will become cations. [p. 8]

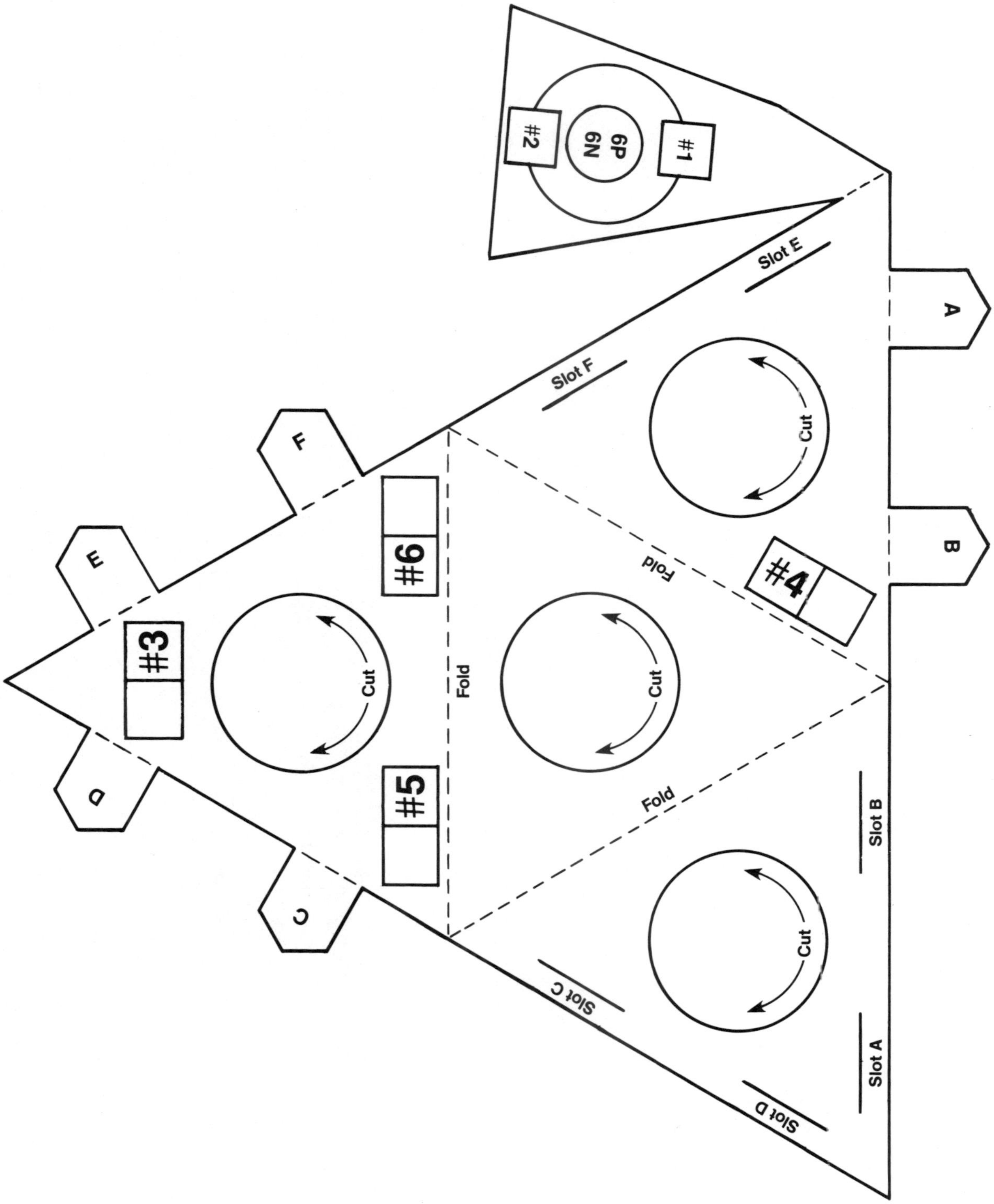

Figure 2–4. Model of the tetrahedral arrangement of electron groups around the carbon nucleus. Directions for assembly: 1) Cut out entire figure. 2) Cut out the 4 circles. 3) Cut the slots for the tabs. 4) Fold on the dotted lines to make a tetrahedron (pyramid shape). 5) Fold the carbon nucleus piece inside the tetrahedron. 6) Fold tabs and fit into slots.

5. Will elements in column VII of the periodic chart tend to gain or lose electrons? How many? Why? What type of ion will they become?

Elements in column VII will tend to gain one electron because they have seven electrons in their valence shell. Because the tendency of all atoms is to mimic the closest inert gas in the periodic table, elements in column VII will find it easier to gain one electron than to lose seven electrons. They will become anions. [p. 8]

6. Why are the inert gases (in column VIII of the periodic chart) always stable?

They are stable because the outer shell (valence shell) of the electron configuration is filled. This is the stable configuration that all atoms want to obtain. Inert gases will never gain or lose electrons. They remain constantly stable with completely filled outer electron shells. [p. 8]

7. What are ions?

Ions are atoms that have gained or lost electrons. They occur when there is a complete transfer of electrons from one atom to another. The gain or loss of electrons by the respective atoms creates an electrical imbalance, giving the atom an overall net electrical charge (– or +). [p. 8]

8. What are cations?

Cations are ions that have *lost* electrons. Because electrons are negatively charged, when an atom loses electrons, there are more positively charged protons present, giving a net positive electrical charge to the atom. *Example*: lithium ion = Li^{+} (lost one electron). [p. 8]

9. What are anions?

Anions are ions that have *gained* electrons. This causes an increase in negatively charged particles within the atom, giving a net negative electrical charge to the atom. *Example*: fluoride ion = F^{-1} (gained one electron). [p. 8]

10. What determines the chemical properties of elements?

The chemical properties of an element depend on the number of electrons in the valence (outer) shell. The tendency of an atom to want to gain or lose electrons determines how it normally reacts with other atoms to form bonds. [p. 8]

11. What are four major bioelements found in biological systems?

Four major bioelements are carbon, hydrogen, nitrogen, and oxygen. [p. 8]

12. How many electrons does hydrogen have available in its valence shell to form bonding sites with other atoms?

Hydrogen has one electron available for bonding with other atoms. It will form one bond in its molecular state. [p. 8]

13. How many electrons does carbon have available in its valence shell to form bonds with other atoms?

Carbon has four electrons available for bonding. It will form four bonds in its molecular state. [p. 8–11]

14. What is a chemical bond?

In general, a chemical bond can be defined as an electrical interaction that links two atoms together. It is achieved by the sharing of a pair of electrons. [p. 11]

15. How many electrons does nitrogen have available in its valence shell to form bonds with other atoms?

Nitrogen has three electrons available for bonding. It will form three bonds in its molecular state. [p. 11]

16. How many electrons does oxygen have available in its valence shell to form bonds with other atoms?

Oxygen has two electrons available for bonding. It will form two bonds in its molecular state. [p. 11]

17. What spatial arrangement do the bioelements tend to form when joined together to form a molecule?

Carbon-containing biomolecules form a tetrahedron. Prime examples include carbon-containing molecules in which carbon is at the center of the tetrahedron with its four bonds at each corner of the tetrahedron. This shape occurs because the electrons available for bonding exist in a tetrahedral configuration around the carbon nucleus. Oxygen-containing biomolecules with oxygen's two unpaired electrons form an inverted V. Nitrogen has three unpaired electrons in a pyramidal arrangement. Because the hydrogen atom has only one bonding electron, it forms linear molecules. [p. 11–12]

CHAPTER 3

THE NATURE OF CHEMICAL BONDS

From the preceeding chapters you learned the concept of electron bonding. You have a visual understanding of electron locations in tetrahedral, pyramidal, and inverted V arrangements for carbon, nitrogen, and oxygen, respectively. Now consider the *types* of bonds that form between two atoms.

When two or more atoms are linked by a chemical bond (a shared pair of electrons), a **molecule** is formed. In contrast to the 106 known types of atoms, millions of types of molecules are known to exist (millions of different combinations of the 106 different types of atoms bonded together). The **molecular weight** of any specific type of molecule is the weight of 1 mole of the molecule, and it represents the combined atomic weights of all the atoms present in that molecule.

A chemical *bond* is defined as the linking together of two atoms by the sharing of an electron pair between the two atoms. As shown in Figure 3–1, three types of bonds are possible. 1) A **nonpolar covalent bond** (top of figure) occurs when the electron pair is equidistant between the nuclei of both atoms. This is the most stable of all chemical bonds and will not break apart in water. 2) An **ionic bond** (bottom of figure) forms when the electron pair is located so close to one of the two nuclei that the chemical bond falls apart when the molecule is placed in water, producing two ions. Water tends to "pull apart" ionic bonds to produce the respective ions. 3) A **polar covalent bond** (middle of figure) exists when the electron pair is not equidistant to both nuclei and at the same time is not so close to one of the two nuclei that the bond will break apart in water. The electron pair is shifted toward one of the two atoms in a polar covalent bond, but the bond will not break apart in water. The bond is called "polar" because the electron pair is shifted to one end or pole of the molecule, and "covalent" because the bond will not break apart in water.

Why and when do these three types of bonds form? Nonpolar covalent bonds form when neither of the two participating atoms in the molecule wants the electron pair more than the other. A good example of this is the bonds that form between carbon and hydrogen. Carbon does not want either to gain or lose electrons (see Figure 2–3). It must lose four electrons to look like helium or gain four electrons to look like neon. Similarly, hydrogen does not care whether it loses its one electron or gains one electron to look like helium. Thus, neither the carbon nor the hydrogen atom holds a greater claim to the electron pair. The result is a stable nonpolar covalent bond between carbon and hydrogen (the electron pair is equidistant between both atoms).

Ionic bonds form when one atom holds a much greater claim to the electron pair than the other atom in the molecule. A good example of an ionic bond is that between lithium (#3 in the periodic table), which wants to lose one electron to look like helium, and fluorine (#9), which needs to gain only one electron to have a completed outer shell and thus look like neon. The molecule lithium fluoride (see Figure 2–2) is held together by an ionic bond. The electron pair shared between these two atoms is so closely held by fluorine that when the lithium fluoride molecule is placed in water, the molecular ionic bond breaks and the entire electron pair goes to fluorine. The fluorine anion (F^-) and the lithium cation (Li^+) are produced when the bond breaks apart in water.

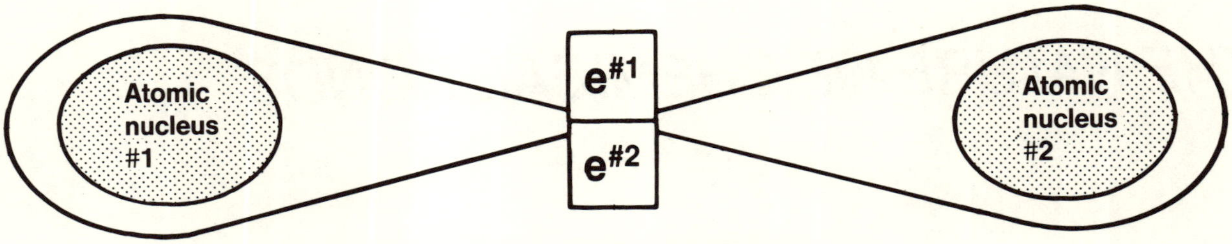

NONPOLAR COVALENT BONDING
(Equal sharing of electron pair)

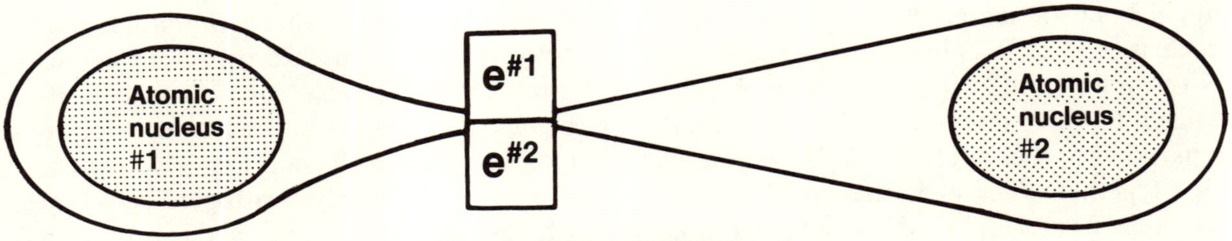

POLAR COVALENT BONDING
(Unequal sharing of electron pair)

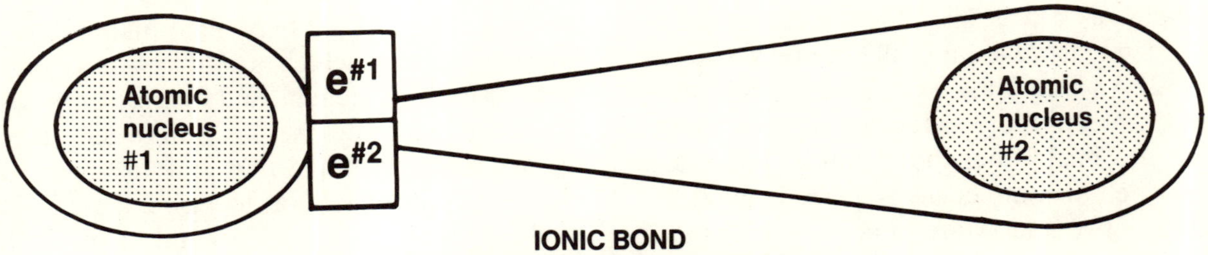

IONIC BOND
(Very unequal sharing of electron pair; bond breaks apart in water)

Figure 3–1. Representation of the three types of chemical bonds. (e#1 = electron from atom #1; e#2 = electron from atom #2)

Polar covalent bonds form when one atom wants the electron pair more than the other atom in the bond, but does not hold the electron pair so tightly that the bond breaks apart in water. The vast majority of molecular bonds that we will study are of the polar covalent type. For example, when oxygen shares two electron pairs with two hydrogen atoms to form a water molecule (Figure 3–2), the electron pairs of each bond are held closer to the oxygen atom. Hydrogen does not care whether it gains or loses an electron, but oxygen does and will hold each electron pair close to its nucleus, but not so close that the bond will break apart in water. This is a very typical example of the types of polar covalent bonds found in biomolecules.

Molecular polarity is the last critical concept in basic chemistry we will discuss. This concept involves the electrical *polarity of polar covalent bonds* and the *tetrahedral spatial arrangement* of those bonds around the bioelement atoms. **Molecular polarity** is a measurement of whether the electron pairs found in a molecule are symmetrical and balanced *or* whether the electron pairs appear to be clustered toward one end (pole) of a molecule.

In the molecule *methane* (CH_4) as seen in Figure 3–3, the carbon atom is at the center of the molecule, with four hydrogen atoms arranged in a *tetrahedral* arrangement around it. Each line connecting the hydrogen and carbon represents an electron pair that is equidistant to both atoms. There is no way of visualizing the molecule so that more electron pairs appear clustered at one end or pole of the molecule. In methane, the electron pairs are symmetrically arranged around the carbon atom. Thus, *methane is not a polar molecule.*

Water (Figure 3–4) is a polar molecule. This phenomenon stems from two facts about water (H_2O): 1) The bonds between hydrogen and oxygen are **polar covalent** because oxygen holds each electron pair closer to its nucleus. 2) The tetrahedral arrangement of the four electron pair spaces around oxygen cause the *two unpaired electrons in the oxygen atom to bond in an inverted V arrangement.* Consequently, the bonds between the two hydrogen atoms and the oxygen atom are also in an inverted V arrange-

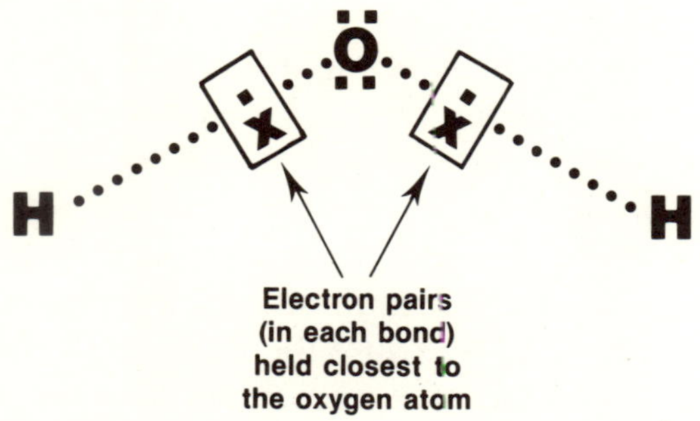

Figure 3–2. Distribution of electron pairs between hydrogen and oxygen in water. ■ = the electrons in the outer electron shell of oxygen atom. ✖ = the electrons in the outer shell of each hydrogen atom.

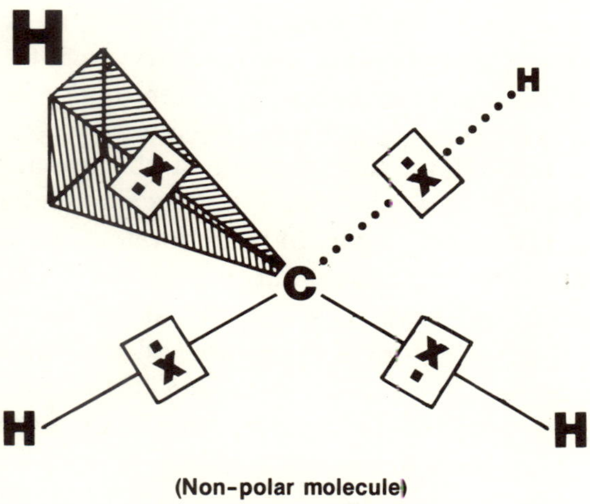

Figure 3–3. The spatial arrangement of bonds found in methane ($-CH_4$). ■ = the electrons found in the outer electron shell of the carbon atom. ✖ = the electrons found in the outer shell of each hydrogen atom.

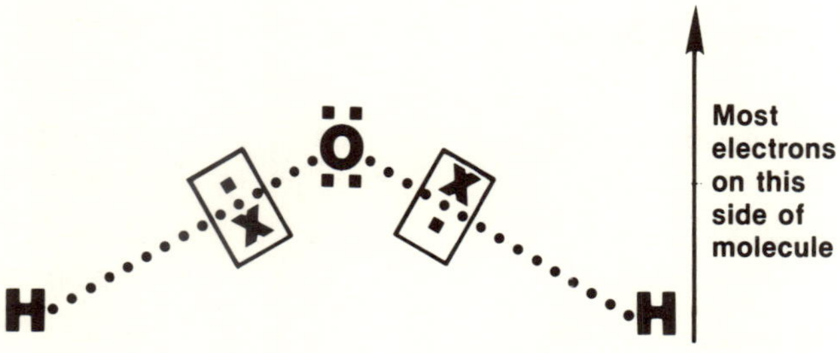

Figure 3–4. Water (H_2O) as a polar molecule. ■ = the electrons in the outer electron shell of oxygen. ✖ = the electrons in the outer shell of each hydrogen atom.

ment. When the entire water molecule is viewed from either the peak of the inverted V or from the two ends of the inverted V, it is clear that *the negatively charged electron pairs tend to cluster around the oxygen end of the molecule* and the hydrogen ends bear a positive charge because of the unequal affinity for the electron pairs in the bond. Because there are more electrons on one side of the molecule than on the other, the *entire water molecule is considered to be a polar molecule*. The polar covalent bonds that form between hydrogen and oxygen are not the only reason for the polarity of the water molecule. If the bonds formed in a linear arrangement rather than in an inverted V, the electron pairs would still appear to be symmetrically clustered around the oxygen atom. However, because of the *tetrahedral spatial arrangement* of the *polar covalent bonds* in water, the polar nature of the entire molecule becomes evident.

To understand the function of the immune system at a molecular level it is critical to understand 1) the polar nature of polar covalent bonds; 2) the tetrahedral spatial arrangement of these bonds in the molecules formed; and 3) the resultant polar nature of these molecules. To summarize (see Table 3–1), *hydrogen* has a single electron available for bonding and usually forms nonpolar covalent bonds because it does not care whether it gains or loses an electron. Hydrogen atoms do not have a preferred location for electron pair bonding. For this reason, hydrogen tends to form nonpolar covalent bonds. An exception to this rule is found when hydrogen atoms bond to oxygen and create **ionic-type bonds** (to be reviewed in Chapter 4—Acids, Bases and the pH Scale). *Carbon* has four electrons available for bonding in its outer shell. The four electrons are arranged in a tetrahedral arrangement around the nucleus. Like hydrogen, carbon does not care whether it gains or loses electrons; nor does it care where the electron pairs are located in a chemical bond. Both hydrogen and carbon tend to form nonpolar covalent bonds, especially when bonded to one another. In contrast, *nitrogen* has three unpaired electrons available for bonding in its outer shell. These three electrons are organized in a pyramidal arrangement below the nucleus (the fourth electron pair position is filled). Nitrogen tends to want to gain electrons and to form polar covalent bonds with other atoms by holding the electron pairs close to its nucleus. *Oxygen* has only two unpaired electrons available for bonding (the other two electron pair positions are filled). These two electron pair spaces are located in an inverted V arrangement below the oxygen atomic nucleus. Because oxygen would like to gain two more electrons, it tends to hold electron pairs close to it, creating polar covalent bonds.

Table 3–1. Bonding Characteristics of the Bioelements.

Name	*Symbol*	*Valence Electrons Available for Bonding*	*How Close Electron Pairs Are Held to Nucleus*	*Types of Bonds*	*Arrangement of Bonding Electrons*
Hydrogen	H	1	Does not care about electron pair position	Nonpolar covalent or ionic (acids)	Linear
Carbon	C	4	Does not care about electron pair position	Nonpolar conalent	Tetrahedral
Nitrogen	N	3	Does want to hold electrons close	Polar covalent	Pyramidal
Oxygen	O	2	Does want to hold electrons close	Polar covalent	Inverted V

Suggested Reading

Ouellette, R. J. *Introduction to General, Organic and Biological Chemistry*. New York: Macmillan, 1984.

Widom, J. M. and S. J. Edelstein. *Chemistry*. San Francisco: Freeman, 1981.

REVIEW QUESTIONS for The Nature of Chemical Bonds

1. What is molecular weight?

Molecular weight is the combined atomic weights of each atom in a molecule. For example, one methane molecule (CH_4) has a molecular weight of 1 gram/mole for each hydrogen (4), and 12 grams/mole for the carbon = 16 grams/mole total. [p. 17]

2. What is a nonpolar covalent bond? Provide an example.

Nonpolar covalent bonds are formed by the equal sharing of electron pairs between two atoms. This occurs because neither of the component atoms wants the electron pair more than the other. This bond will not break apart in water. *Example*: Bonds between hydrogen and carbon (as in methane (CH_4)) are nonpolar covalent bonds. [p. 17]

3. What is a polar covalent bond? Provide an example.

Polar covalent bonds are formed when unequal sharing of electron pairs occurs between two atoms, but the bond will not break apart in water. One atom attracts the electron pair more vigorously than the other atom; thus, the electron pair spends more time at one end (pole) of the bond than at the other.
Example: Water (H_2O) has polar covalent bonds:

The oxygen atom wants each electron pair more than the hydrogens want them. [p. 17]

4. What is an ionic bond? Provide an example.

Ionic bonds are extreme examples of polar bonds. In ionic bonds, the electron pair is held extremely close to one of the atoms. The distinguishing difference between ionic and polar covalent bonds is that ionic bonds break apart in water to form ions.
Example: Lithium fluoride (LiF) = (Li :F). The electron pair sits so close to the fluoride atom that the bond breaks apart in water and fluoride keeps the electron pair. Thus, the cation Li^+ and the anion F^- are formed. [p. 17]

5. What produces the polar nature of certain molecules?

The polar nature of certain molecules occurs when the bonds in the molecule are polar and arranged in a tetrahedral pyramidal or inverted V spatial arrangement. [p. 17]

6. Why is the shape of a water molecule like an inverted V?

The inverted V shape of a water molecule results from the inverted V shape of the two electrons available for bonding around the oxygen atom. The two hydrogens must bond at the sites of the two available electrons found in an inverted V arrangement around oxygen.

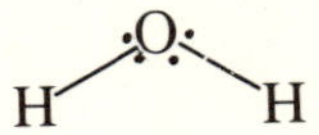

[p. 19]

7. Water has a neutral overall charge but is a polar molecule. What are the charges of each pole of the water molecule? Why?

The two hydrogen ends of the inverted V of the water molecule bear a positive charge because of the unequal affinity of oxygen and hydrogen for the electron pairs in the bonds. Oxygen wants to hold the electron pairs more closely than does each hydrogen. Thus, the hydrogen electrons stay closer to the oxygen than to their respective hydrogens, taking their negative charge to the apex of the inverted V which has a more negative charge because all the electrons are positioned here. [p. 20]

CHAPTER 4

ACIDS, BASES, AND THE pH SCALE

Hydrogen is the only bioelement that frequently forms ionic bonds because it bonds so often with oxygen, an atom with an intense desire for the electron pair. When placed in water, hydrogen-oxygen molecules tend to release free hydrogen ions. The hydrogen atom stripped of its only electron becomes the hydrogen ion H^+. A hydrogen ion is equivalent to **acid**. Molecules that release free hydrogen ion when dropped in water are also known as acids. Molecules that accept free hydrogen ions (H^+) are known as **bases**. Acids release free hydrogen ions; bases are capable of absorbing or accepting hydrogen ions (removing them from solution).

The **pH scale** was developed to measure the strengths of acids and bases. The scale ranges from 0 to 14 (Figure 4–1). In the middle of the scale is pH 7, which is the neutral pH value of the acidity of water. From pH 7 to pH 0, the acidity of a solution (the concentration of free hydrogen ions) increases; pH 0 is the strongest acid possible. In contrast, from pH 7 to pH 14, the concentration of free hydrogen ions drops even lower than the concentration of H^+ found in water; thus, a base must be present in the solution that is absorbing (neutralizing) free hydrogen ions. Basic solutions are also known as **alkaline solutions**. At the far end of the pH scale is pH 14, the strongest possible base; this substance will literally rip free hydrogen ions (absorb them) from just about any molecule that contains hydrogen.

Many of the biomolecules presented in subsequent chapters have acidic components (such as nucleic acids and amino acids). In addition, it is important to remember that most organ systems of the human body (including the immune system) function best at a specific pH of 7.4. Any change in body pH from 7.4 (either more basic or more acidic) could result in serious impairment of body function.

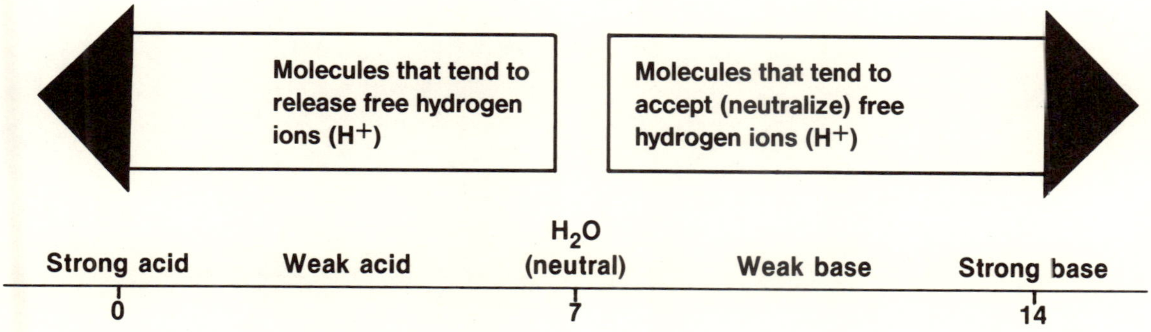

Figure 4–1. The pH scale.

Suggested Reading

Brody, J. E. and G. E. Humiston. *General Chemistry, Principles and Structure*. 3rd ed. New York: Wiley, 1982.

Wingrove, A. S. *Organic Chemistry*. New York: Harper & Row, 1981.

REVIEW QUESTIONS for Acids, Bases, and The pH Scale

1. What is an acid?

An acid is any substance that tends to donate, or release, hydrogen ions (H^+). This tendency to release free hydrogen ions into solution causes an increase in the hydrogen ion concentration (the acidity) of the solution. [p. 23]

2. What is a base?

A base is any substance that tends to accept hydrogen ions from solution. This tendency to gain free hydrogen ions from a solution causes a decrease in the hydrogen ion concentration of that solution. Basic solutions are also known as alkaline solutions. [p. 23]

3. Describe the pH scale.

The pH scale is a measure of relative hydrogen ion concentration, based on a scale of 0 to 14, with 7 being neutral. Any values below 7 denote an acidic solution, while values increasing above 7 denote an increasingly basic (alkaline) solution. pH 7 is the acidity of water. [p. 23]

4. What does the pH of a solution denote?

The pH of a solution is a measure of its acidity or alkalinity. The concentration of hydrogen ions in the solution determines its degree of acidity or alkalinity. The higher the hydrogen ion concentration, the lower the pH value, and vice versa. [p. 23]

CHAPTER 5

PROTEINS: STRUCTURE AND FUNCTION

In the next four chapters we will review how the four principal bioelements form **biomolecules**. There are four principal types of biomolecules: 1) **proteins**, 2) **lipids**, 3) **carbohydrates** (including starches and sugars), and 4) **nucleic acids** (DNA and RNA). It is not essential to memorize scientific terms or formulas for the biomolecules; rather, try to see "in your mind's eye" the actual three-dimensional structure of these molecules. To do this, have a good three-dimensional visualization in mind of the four *bioelements*—hydrogen, carbon, nitrogen, and oxygen. Please return to the previous chapters if uncertainties regarding the following concepts arise: the four bioelements; the three types of bonds they form; the tetrahedral spatial arrangement of their bonds; and the chemical basis for polar molecules.

The biomolecules are made of certain component subunits that recur over and over again in many different types of biomolecules, as shown in Figure 5–1. For example, an **–OH group** attached (bonded) to a carbon atom that does *not* have any other **double bonds** to oxygen is an **alcohol** or **hydroxyl** group. A double bond is 2 pairs of shared electrons, represented by a double line, such as C=O. An –OH group attached to a carbon which also is attached to another oxygen by a double bond is a

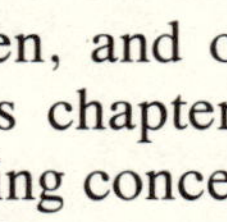

carboxylic acid group. When nitrogen is attached to two hydrogens

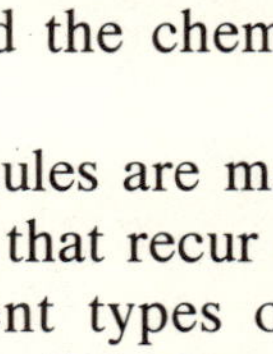

it is an **amino group**.

A phosphorus connected to four oxygens

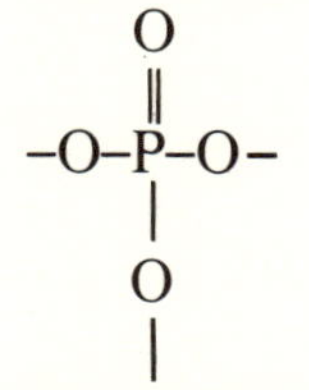

is a **phosphate group.** These groups represent four major types of subunits found in biomolecules.

A *chemical bond* represents a pair of electrons shared between two atoms. In the subsequent drawings, a chemical bond (a shared electron pair) is represented by a single line drawn between two atoms; a double line (*double bond*) represents *two pairs of shared electrons*.

Proteins, also known as polypeptides, are chains of connecting subunits kown as *amino acids*. There are 20 common amino acids. All 20 amino acids bear the same basic structure, as shown in Figure 5–2. Please note the amino acid structure and components: 1) A **central carbon** atom is joined to an $-NH_2$ group on the left side which is known as an **amino group**. 2) A –COOH group is joined to the central carbon on the right side and is known as a **carboxylic acid group.** 3) A **single hydrogen** is joined at the top. 4) An **R group** is joined to the central carbon at the bottom. The **R** represents a *replacement group*. The *R group is different in each of the 20 amino acids*. Thus, a simple amino acid might have only a $-CH_3$ group where the R group sits, such as alanine. Other amino acids might have complicated ring-like hydrocarbon structures for the R group, such as phenylalanine. Figure 5–3 shows a few examples.

When reviewing chemical diagrams, please keep three very important facts in mind: 1) The molecules are drawn in the simple two-dimen-

Subunit Group	Example
-OH Hydroxyl (alcohol) group	
-COOH Carboxylic acid group	
$-NH_2$ Amino group	
$-H_2PO_4$ Phosphate group	

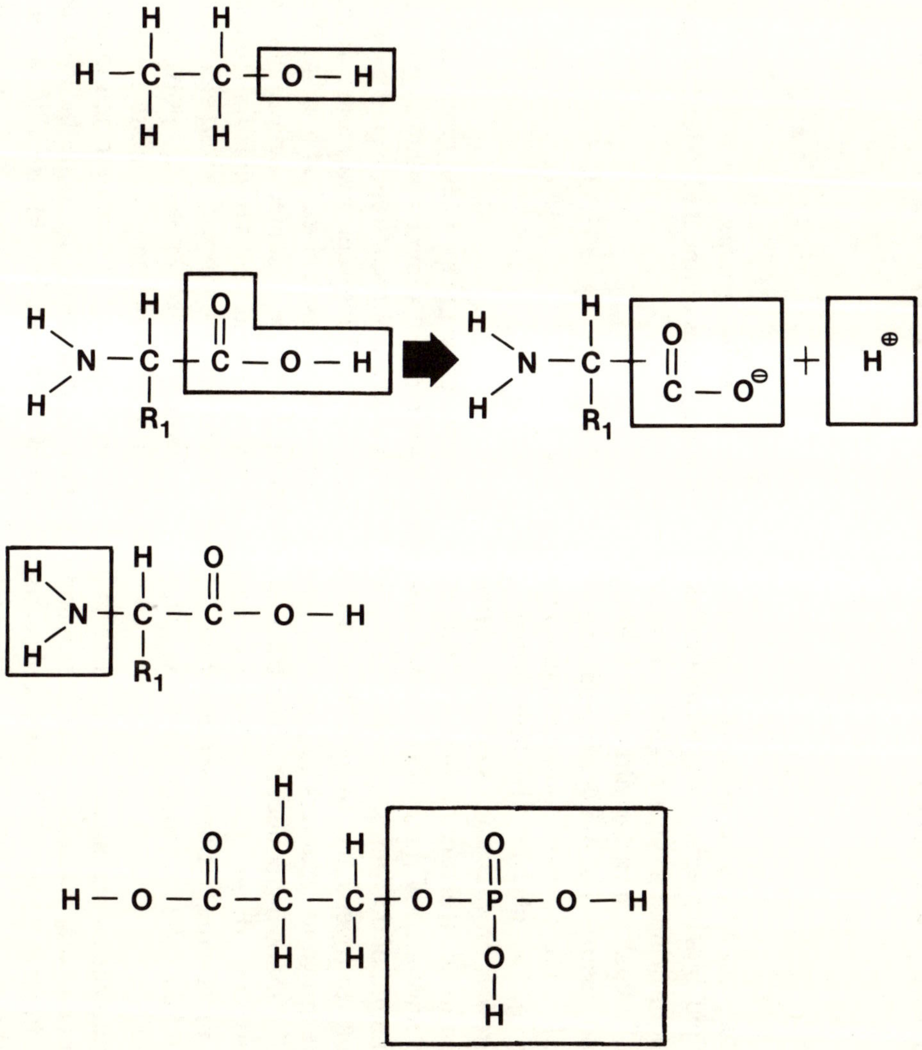

Figure 5–1. Four major types of subunits on biomolecules.

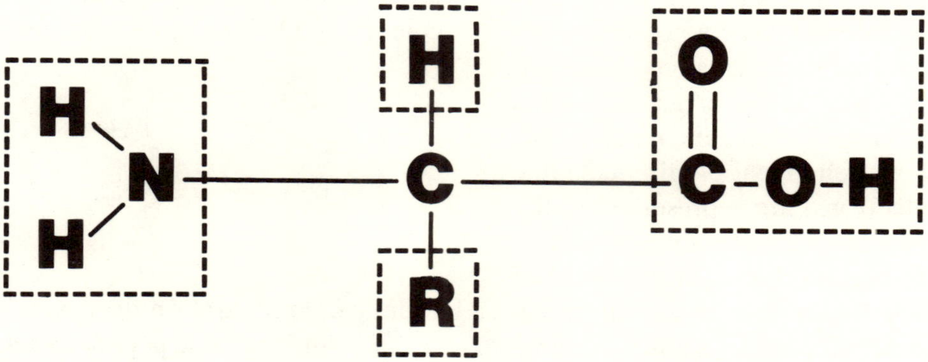

Figure 5–2. Basic structure of an amino acid.

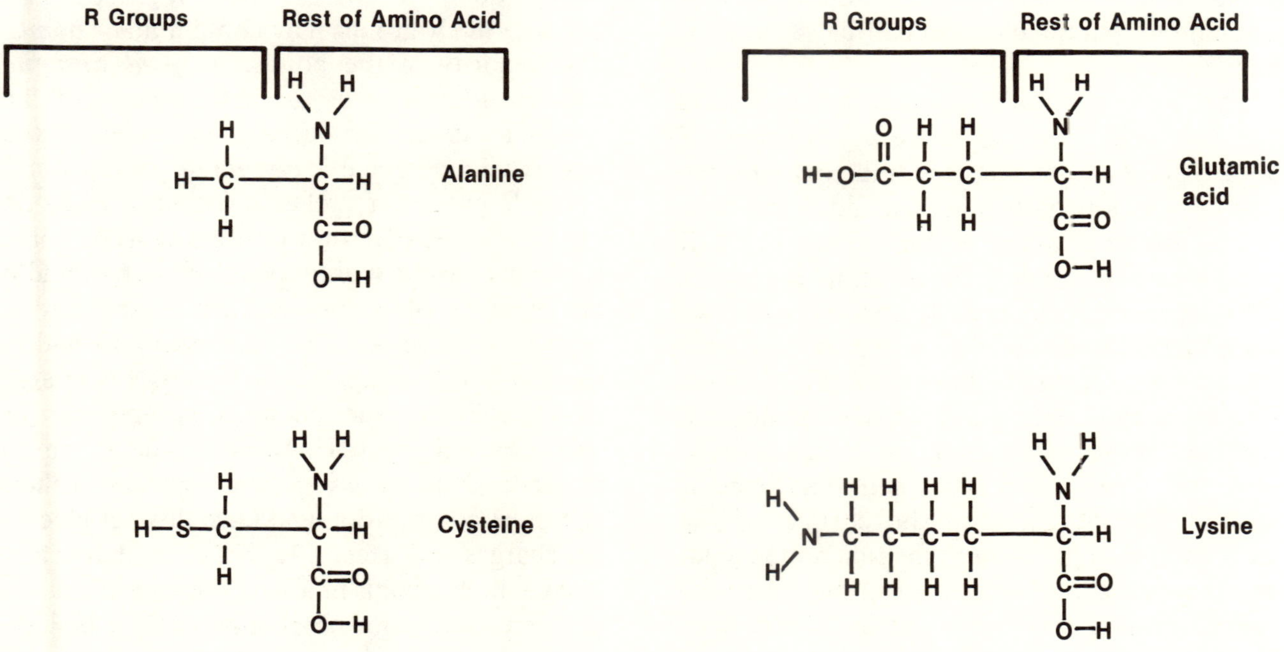

Figure 5–3. Examples of types of R groups on four different amino acids.

sional form discussed in Chapter 2. Remember that the bonds between atoms are not 90° bonds as they appear in the two-dimensional diagram, but are actually 110° bonds arranged in the tetrahedral structure. 2) The chemical bonds between atoms (one chemical bond equals one shared pair of electrons) are represented in the diagrams by a single line between the atomic symbols (one line equals one shared pair of electrons). Double bonds exist in certain molecules (for example, C = O); again, a double bond simply indicates that two pairs of electrons are shared between the two atoms. 3) Remember that each bond represented in the diagram can be one of three types—nonpolar covalent, ionic, or polar covalent. In molecules such as the amino acids, all three types of bonds are represented. The top bond between carbon and the solitary hydrogen is a nonpolar covalent bond because neither atom has a preference for where the electron pair is located. The bond between the oxygen and hydrogen in the carboxylic acid group (–COOH) is ionic because when that bond is placed in water, it dissociates to release a hydrogen ion (H^+) (acid; reviewed in Chapter 4). The bonds between carbon and oxygen or the bonds between carbon and nitrogen tend to be polar covalent bonds because nitrogen and oxygen tend to pull the electron pair closer to their nucleus.

The basic structure of amino acids involve two more critical points: 1) the way amino acids hook together by means of peptide bond formation to form long polypeptides, and 2) the most distinguishing features of the amino acid's R group (the *size* and the *polarity* of the R groups). The formation of the peptide bond between two amino acids, and thus the formation of a *polypeptide*, is rather straightforward (Figure 5–4). The carboxylic acid group of one amino acid approaches the amino group of a second amino acid and a new bond is formed. The bond is formed directly between the carbon of the carboxylic acid group from the first amino acid, and the nitrogen of the amino group from the second amino acid. One of the hydrogens from the amino group and the OH part of the acid group come together to form a separate molecule of H_2O. Any time you see the

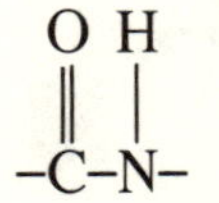

chemical configuration displayed in Figure 5–4, you are looking at a **peptide bond**. By forming peptide bonds with one another, large numbers of single amino acids can hook together to form a large *polypeptide*. A polypeptide can be as short as three or four amino acids or as long as thousands of amino acids.

As mentioned previously, the only distinctive part of each amino acid is the R group that it possesses. It can be very small, like a $-CH_3$ group (as found in alanine), or substantially larger (as found in lysine). There are two points about R groups that are easy to remember: 1) There are 20 different types of R groups known; thus, at least 20 different types of "common" amino acids (commonly found in proteins) are known. 2) The most important characteristics about each R group are the *size* and *charge* (polarity) that they possess. The charges on the R groups differ because the R groups may contain *polar bonds*. The polarity of the bonds, *coupled with the tetrahedral nature* of the arrangement of the bonds in space, produces *polar areas* of the amino acid molecule *in certain of the R groups*. Some R groups are relatively neutral (they do not have a negative or a positive charge), some R groups have a slightly positive charge, and a fair number of R groups have a very strong negative charge. It is not necessary to understand which R groups have which type of charge or to know the exact chemical composition or size of each R group. However, it is important to understand that *R groups are different* in their chemical composition and have distinct electrical charges and sizes. The electrical charge and size of the R groups in a long polypeptide chain account for a major proportion of their biological activity. In Figure 5–5 this concept is com-

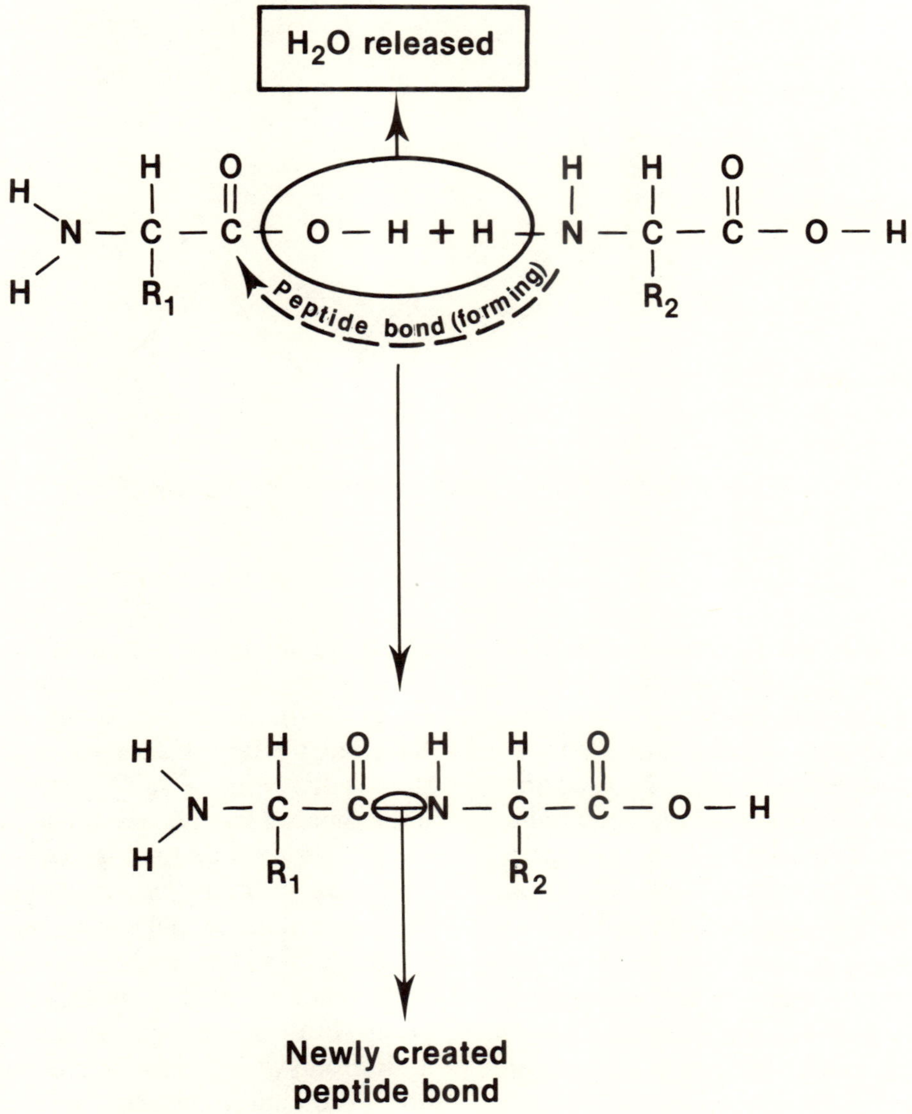

Figure 5–4. Formation of a peptide bond.

pared with the teeth on a key: if the teeth are not in exactly the right position and of the right size, they will not turn the lock chambers. Similarly, the charges that exist on the R groups of a long polypeptide chain must be in exactly the right sequence to produce certain biological activities. The peptide bonds between the amino and carboxylic acid groups form the backbone of the key, and the R groups of the amino acids project outward like the teeth of a key. The differences in the size and shape of the teeth of a key are analogous to the differences in the sizes and electrical charges (polarity) of the different R groups of the sequence of amino acids in any given protein.

The number of possible different polypeptides is enormous. At each amino acid site there can be 1 of 20 different amino acids. Similarly,

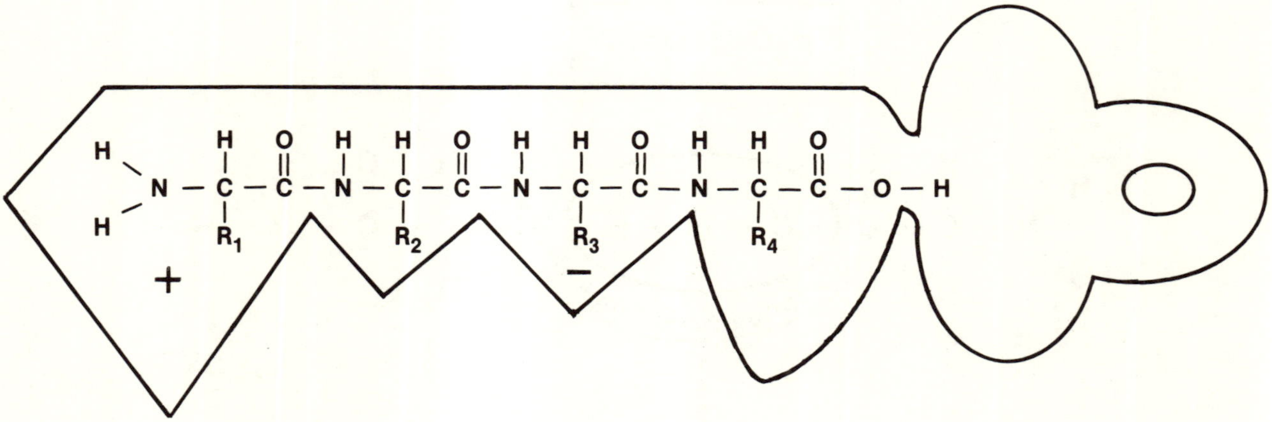

Figure 5–5. Analogy between a short peptide and a key.

at the next amino acid site, another 20 possibilities exist, and so on. The total number of different polypeptides that can be created in a peptide 100 amino acids long, with at least 20 amino acids possible at each site, is 20 × 20 × 20 and so on for 100 multiplications (a very large number!). As mentioned previously, some polypeptides are thousands of amino acids long; the total number of different types of proteins known is mind-boggling.

The infinity variety of amino acid sequences that can exist in a peptide, and thus the variety of R group sequences with their respective sizes and charges, is only part of the biological story of proteins and their activity. Biochemists have analyzed protein structure at four levels: primary, secondary, tertiary and quaternary. **Primary structure** is simply the amino acid sequence of a protein as illustrated in Figure 5–6. The primary structure of a protein can be described by simply citing a list of the amino acids in that protein in order. However, a fascinating scientific fact is that many polypeptides tend to instantly *coil upon themselves*, much like a "slinky." This coiling, as shown in Figure 5–6, is known as the **alpha helix configuration** and occurs because of electrical interactions between polar portions surrounding each peptide bond. Because the peptide bonds are regularly spaced between each amino acid in the protein, these electrical attraction sites tend to cause the protein to change immediately from its primary structure into a coiled-spring **secondary structure**. The **tertiary structure** of a protein refers to the tendency of certain proteins to fold back upon themselves once the alpha helix is formed, much like a slinky folding back upon itself. A "globular structure" is formed by the folding. This three-dimensional configuration of the polypeptide chain is created by electrical attractions between different R groups. For example, an R group with a positive charge may be attracted to an R group with a negative charge much further down the chain, causing the entire alpha helix to distort and fold back upon itself. However, the most obvious force that causes the protein to assume a three-dimensional or *tertiary structure* is a unique type of bond known as the **disulfide bond**. A disulfide bond forms between two cysteine amino acids. Cysteine is one of the 20 common amino acids previously described; its entire chemical structure, including its **sulfur-containing R group**, is shown in Figure 5–3. The sulfur from the R group of one cysteine easily forms a *nonpolar covalent bond* with the sulfur from any other cysteine R group in the polypeptide chain, and a *disulfide bond* is formed. The disulfide bond, compared with the other R group interactions, is a *nonpolar covalent bond*, not merely an electrical attraction. The fourth level

Primary structure

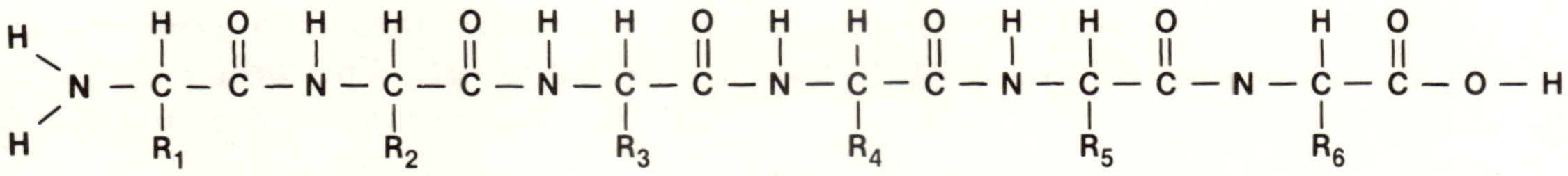

Secondary structure

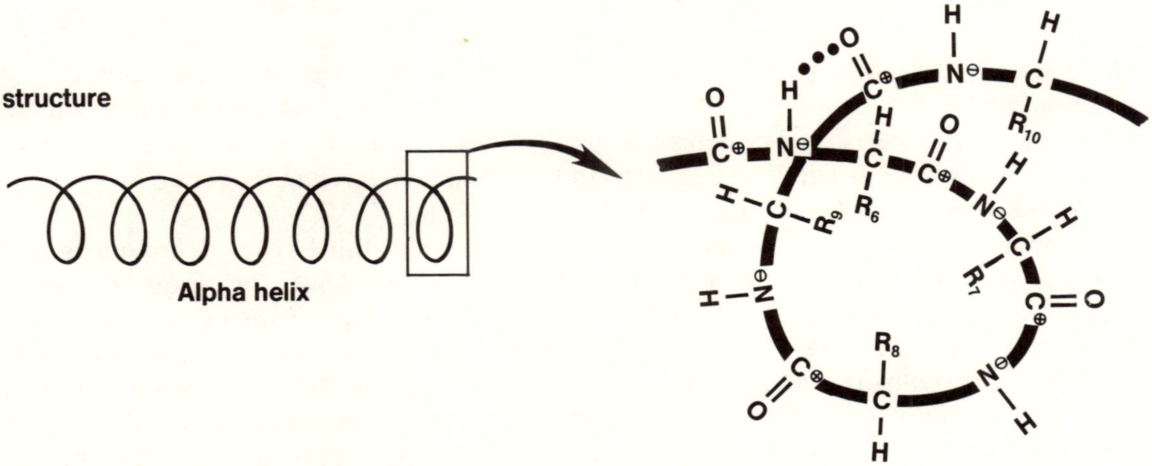

Tertiary structure

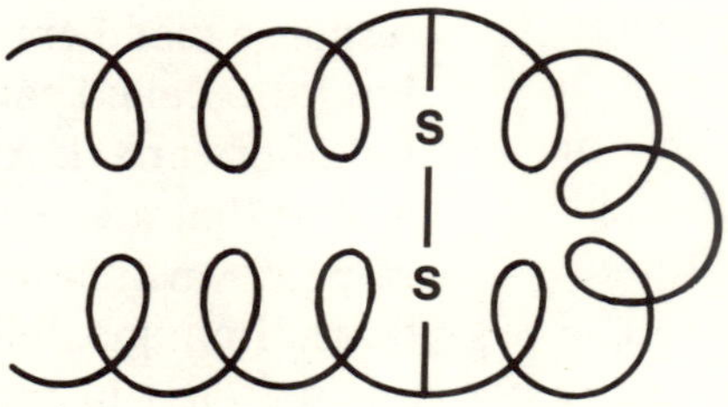

Quaternary structure

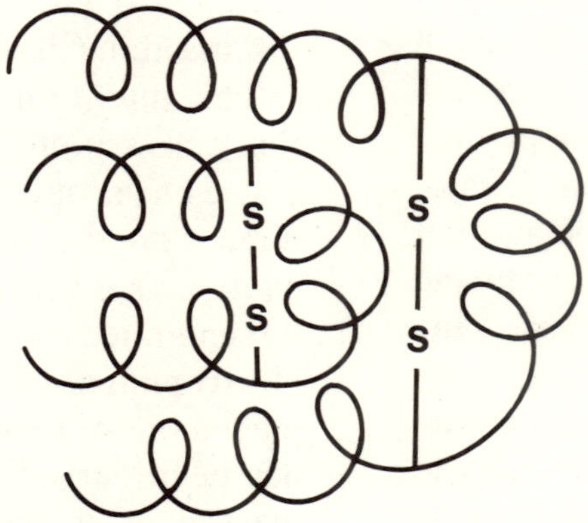

Figure 5–6. Primary, secondary, tertiary, and quaternary structure of peptides.

of structure, or **quaternary structure**, refers to the way that *two or more* polypeptides can be electrically attracted to one another. Two proteins can be physically associated with one another in space, without being covalently bonded to one another (see Figure 5–3).

In review, protein *primary structure* is simply a literal citation of the order of the amino acids in that protein. The *secondary structure* of a protein is the alpha helix configuration that most proteins assume due to the electrical interactions between the polar portions surrounding each peptide bond. The globular, three-dimensional or *tertiary structure* of proteins is caused by electrical attractions between R groups and, most importantly, by the formation of disulfide bonds between two different cysteines on the same polypeptide chain. *Quaternary structure* simply refers to the association (electrical attraction) of two or more polypeptides in space.

Proteins are absolutely critical components for life. Proteins perform three distinct types of functions: 1) structural, 2) enzymatic, and 3) others. As *structural* proteins, certain long polypeptides (such as collagen) are excellent for forming a supportive framework for living tissues. Most of the resistance that you feel when you cut through a piece of meat is, in fact, the protein framework that cells live on and are composed of. The structural proteins tend to be relatively inert; once synthesized, they remain unchanged unless some tissue damage occurs.

Enzymes are specific proteins that **catalyze** or promote certain types of chemical reactions. It is critical to understand what enzymes are and how they work. In the formation of the peptide bond, the amino end of one amino acid must approach the carboxylic acid end of another amino acid in order for water to be cleaved and a peptide bond to be created. Ordinarily, the addition of a certain amount of energy is required for the reaction to occur. For example, when starting a fire you must first add energy to the wood in the form of a lighted match in order for the reaction to proceed on its own. The added energy brings the molecules (reactants) close enough together for the bonds to form and the reaction to proceed. The purpose of enzymes is to bring two reactants together physically in such a way that 1) much less energy has to be added to the system to get bond formation, and 2) the reaction can thus proceed *much more rapidly*. The formation of a peptide bond with and without an enzyme is shown in Figure 5–7. In summary, *enzymes* are a type of nonstructural protein that catalyze (promote) specific types of reactions. For just about every type of metabolic reaction that occurs in the human body, there is a specific enzyme that catalyzes that reaction. Each cell regulates the speed with which the various metabolic reactions occur by regulating the amount of the specific enzyme required for that reaction in the cell.

The third type of protein is categorized as "other." This *other* group of proteins serves a mixed bag of distinct functions; many are of particular interest to immunologists. One such protein is the oxygen-binding protein **hemoglobin** that exists in red blood cells. The proteins that we will study in depth include: 1) **biological response modifiers** (BRM) and 2) **immunoglobulins** (also called **antibodies**). Biological response modifiers are short polypeptide signals or hormones that are secreted by one cell in order to cause downstream cells to perform specific functions. Immunoglobulins are polypeptides that are secreted in immune system cells which in turn are capable of binding to and neutralizing specific molecules that might invade the body. These two fascinating groups of proteins are discussed in Chapters 14 and 24.

The many different polypeptides (proteins) that cells secrete can be separated into different classes by a variety of different laboratory techniques on the basis of their overall size and charge. One way in which protein mixtures can be separated is a technique known as **protein electrophoresis**. This technique involves the placement of a protein mixture in a trough that has been carved into a thin film of gelatinous material, as shown in Figure 5–8. As an electrical current is passed through the film, the various protein species move through the gel on the basis of the net charge of all the R groups on each polypeptide. The proteins with the greatest net

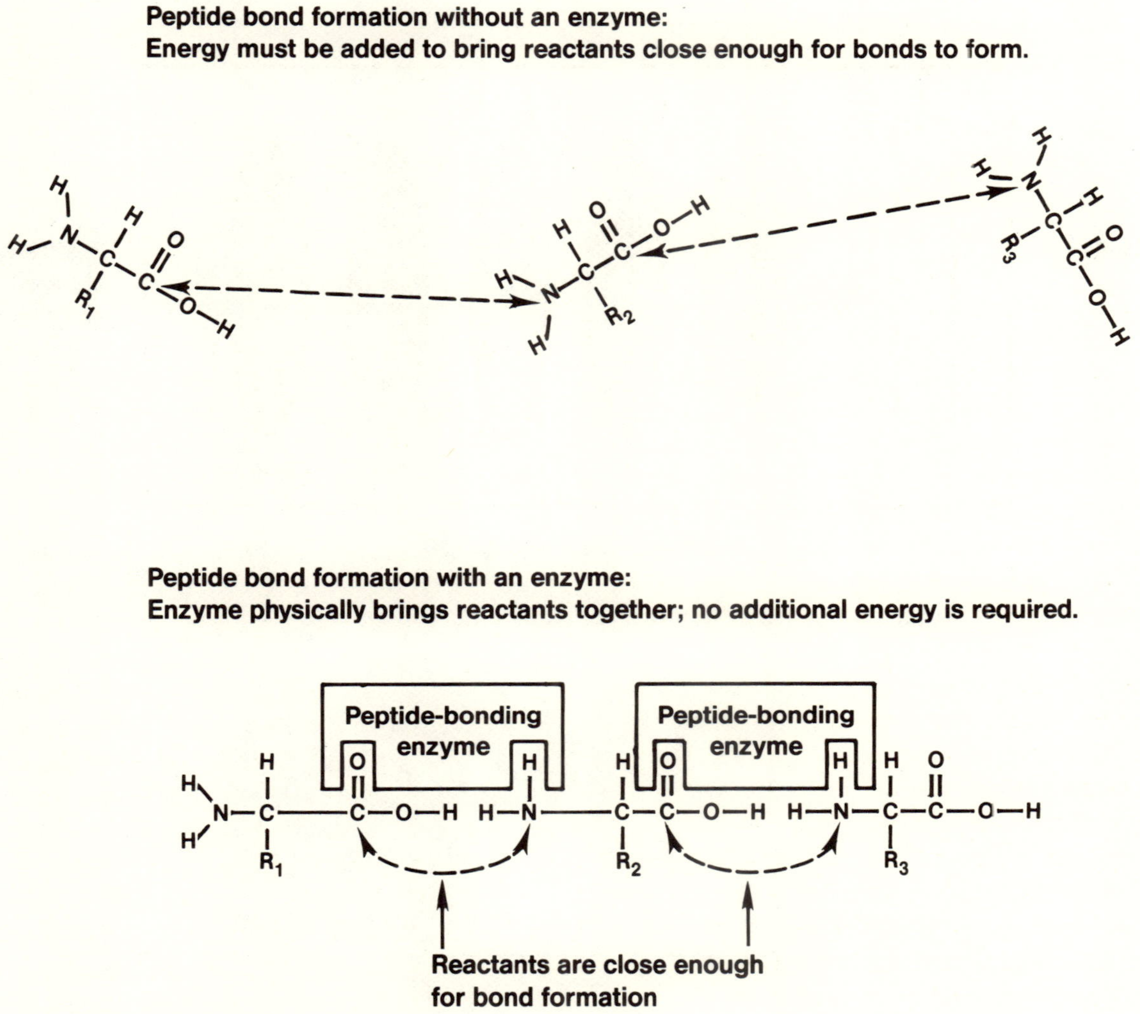

Figure 5–7. Peptide bond formation with and without an enzyme.

negative charge move farthest toward the positive end of the plate. This technique allows the protein mixture found in the human bloodstream to be separated by the electrical charge, and five major groups of proteins can be obtained: 1) **albumin**, 2) **alpha$_1$** (α_1) proteins, 3) **alpha$_2$** (α_2) proteins, 4) **beta** (β) proteins, and 5) **gamma** (γ) proteins. When plotted on a graph according to the *amount* of protein in each group, the representative peaks obtained by protein electrophoresis can appear as in Figure 5–9. The types of proteins that can be found in each of these peaks include the following:

1) Albumin peak—albumin (large proteins found in the bloodstream)
2) α_1 peak—α_1 lipoprotein (proteins to which fats bind) and others
3) α_2 peak—haptoglobin (proteins of the bloodstream that bind to the breakdown products of destroyed red blood cells) and others
4) β peak—complement proteins (certain immunologic proteins to be discussed in Chapter 19) and others
5) γ peak—most immunoglobulin proteins (antibodies, to be discussed in Chapter 14)

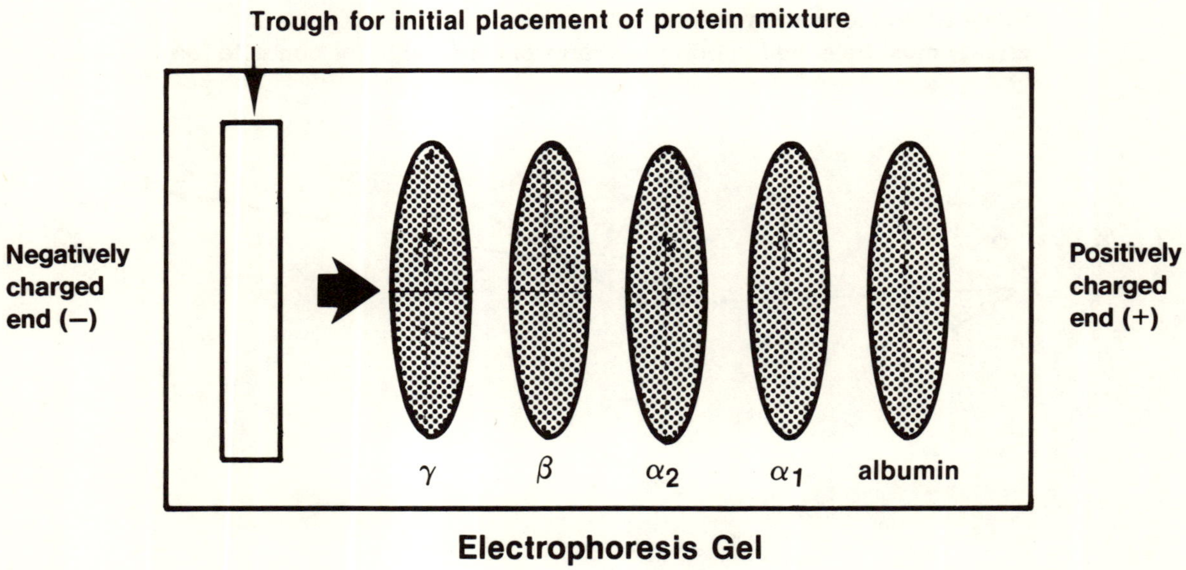

Figure 5–8. Electrophoresis technique for separating proteins.

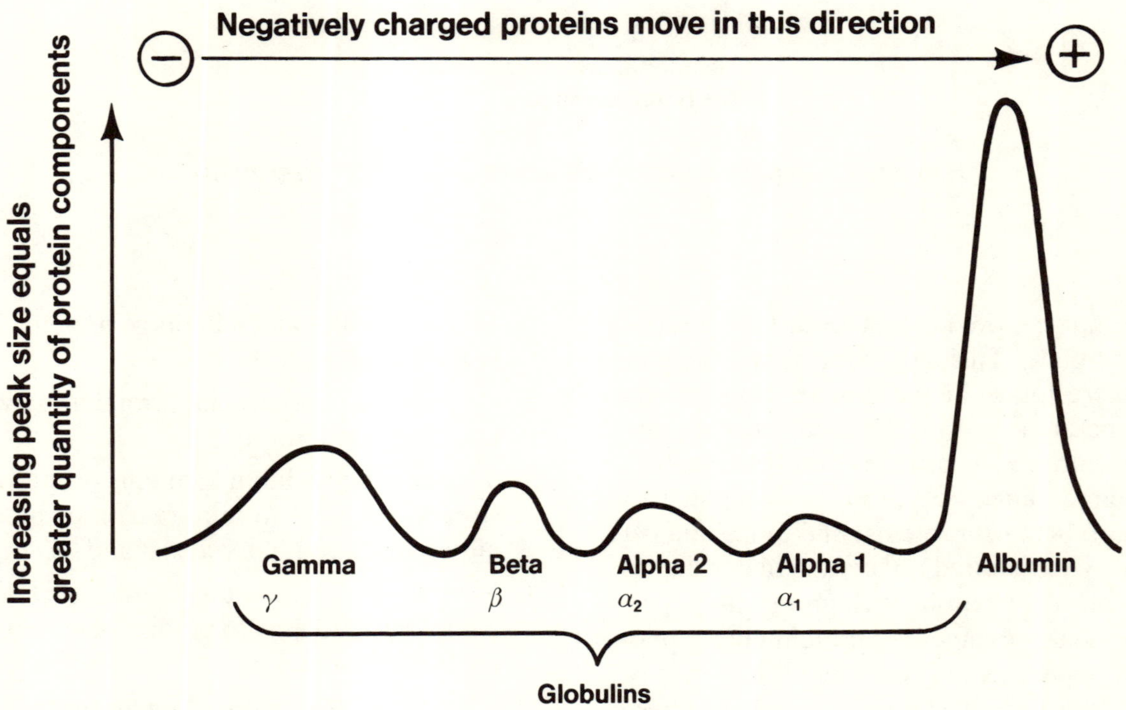

Figure 5–9. Protein peaks obtained by protein electrophoresis of human serum.

Suggested Reading

Dickerson, R. E. and I. Geis. *The Structure and Action of Proteins*. Menlo Park, CA: Benjamin/Cummings, 1969.

Lehninger, A. L. *Principles of Biochemistry*, 8th ed. New York: Worth, 1982.

REVIEW QUESTIONS for Proteins: Structure and Function

1. What are the four major types of biomolecules?

The major biomolecules are proteins, lipids, carbohydrates, and the nucleic acids (RNA and DNA). [p. 25]

2. What are the building blocks of proteins?

Amino acids are the structural building blocks of proteins. [p. 25]

3. Draw the general structure of an amino acid?

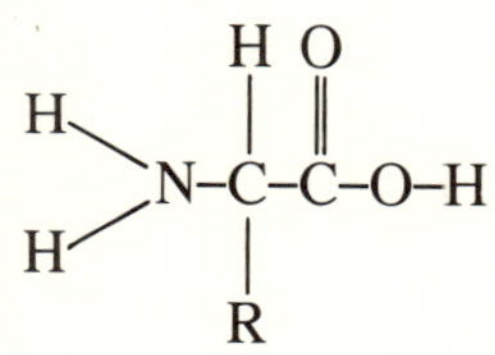

[p. 25]

4. How many types of amino acids are there:

There are 20 common amino acids. [p. 25]

5. How are amino acids similar to each other?

They all have four structural properties in common, that is, an amino group ($-NH_2$), a carboxylic acid group (–COOH), and a solitary hydrogen attached to the central carbon of the molecule. [p. 25]

6. How do amino acids differ from each other?

All amino acids possess a central carbon, an amino group ($-NH_2$), a carboxylic acid group (–COOH), and a solitary hydrogen. The last attachment group to the central carbon is called the R or replacement group side chain. The R groups are different structures from one amino acid to the next, giving the amino acids their individual properties. [p. 28]

7. What are the properties of the R groups that give them their functional differences?

The different sizes and electrical charges from one R group to the next give each R group its functional difference, thus making each amino acid behave differently. [p. 28]

8. What is a polypeptide?

A polypeptide is a sequence of amino acids joined by peptide bonds. [p. 28]

9. How are proteins formed?

The formation of proteins involves a chemical reaction whereby individual amino acids are linked through the formation of a peptide bond. [p. 28]

10. Where is the peptide bond located?

The peptide bond occurs between the carboxylic acid group of one amino acid and the amino group of another. A molecule of water is also formed and released through this reaction. [p. 28]

11. Draw the chemical reaction that occurs between two amino acids to form a protein.

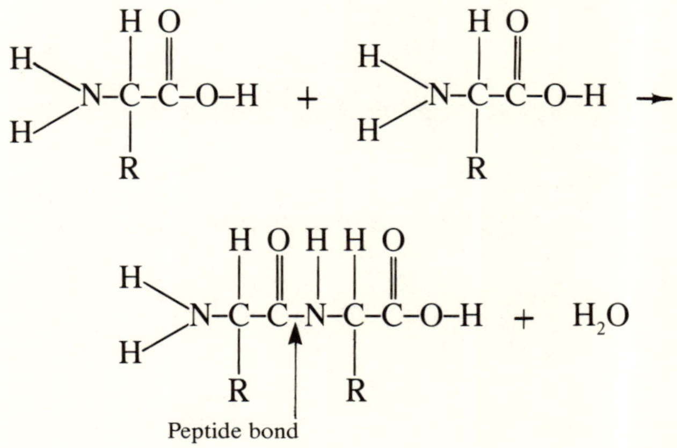

[p. 29]

12. What is the primary structure of a polypeptide?

The primary structure of a protein chain considers only the specific amino acid sequence listing in that protein chain. [p. 30]

13. What is the secondary structure of a polypeptide and why does it occur?

The secondary structure takes into consideration the fact that most proteins do not occur as straight chains but are, in fact, coiled into a regular repeating pattern known as an alpha helix. This pattern occurs because of the electrical attractions between the polar portions surrounding the peptide bonds of neighboring amino acids. [p. 30]

14. Draw an alpha helix.

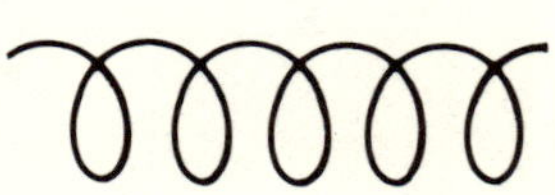

[p. 30]

15. What is the tertiary structure of a polypeptide and why does it occur?

The tertiary structure is the three-dimensional configuration of a protein chain. Two forces affect the tertiary structure of a protein: 1) electrical attractions between R groups can distort the alpha helix structure, 2) covalent bonds form between the sulfur-containing R groups on the amino acid cysteine. Cysteines on different ends of the protein can fuse their R groups to form covalent disulfide bonds. These disulfide bonds distort the protein alpha helix into a three-dimensional globular structure. [p. 30]

16. What does quaternary protein structure refer to?

Quaternary structure refers to the association (electrical attraction) of two or more polypeptides in space. [p. 32]

17. What are three types of proteins and what are their functions?

1) *Structural* proteins form the supportive meshwork for tissues.
2) *Enzymes* catalyze (promote) chemical reactions.
3) *"Other"* proteins function in oxygen-binding (hemoglobin), act as polypeptide signals (hormones, BRM), and are immunoglobulins.

[p. 32]

18. What are enzymes? How do they work?

Enzymes are proteins that catalzye (promote) certain types of chemical reactions. They lower the amount of energy required to make a reaction proceed by physically bringing the reactants together so bonds can form. [p. 32]

19. What is protein electrophoresis?

Protein electrophoresis is a laboratory technique whereby the various polypeptide components of a protein mixture can be separated on the basis of their overall electrical charge. [p. 32]

20. What factor is involved in the movement of the various protein components when a current is passed through them:

The net charge of the polypeptide. [p. 33]

21. In electrophoresis, which proteins move the farthest toward the positive end of the plate? Why?

Proteins that have a greater negative net charge move the farthest. They move the farthest because the positive charge at the end of the plate attracts the protein, causing it to travel through the gel. [p. 33]

22. What are the five major protein groups found in human serum that can be separated by protein electrophoresis?

The five groups are albumin, $alpha_1$, $alpha_2$, beta, and gamma proteins. Human immunoglobulins are in the gamma peak; complement proteins are in the beta peak. [p. 33]

CHAPTER 6

LIPIDS

Lipids are found in many parts of the human body and are integral parts of each living cell. Lipids are classified into three chemical groups: the neutral fats, the phospholipids, and the steroids. All lipids have in common the property that they will not mix with water; that is, they tend to float on top of water much like an oil slick.

Neutral fats are the most common lipids in the body. As shown in Figure 6–1, neutral fats are composed of subunits known as fatty acids, which are attached to a glycerol "backbone." **Fatty acids** are long chains of carbons and hydrogens bonded together (usually 14 to 22 carbons long) that have a very nonpolar $-CH_3$ group on one end and a polar carboxylic acid group ($-COOH$) on the other end. As shown in Figure 6–1, three fatty acids can bond to a glycerol molecule with ester bonds (bonds linking glycerol and fatty acids) to form a molecule known as a **triglyceride** or neutral fat. The word triglyceride indicates the exact chemical composition of this molecule: three fatty acids joined to a glycerol backbone. The major purpose of the neutral lipids in the body is to store energy. Triglycerides can be acted upon by specific enzymes that break down their energy-rich bonds and thus can be used as an energy source for the cells of the body.

Phospholipids are similar in structure to triglycerides, except that one of the three fatty acid chains has been removed from the glycerol backbone and replaced by a very polar phosphate group (PO_4). The PO_4 group sticks out from the glycerol backbone in the opposite direction from the fatty acid chains, as shown in

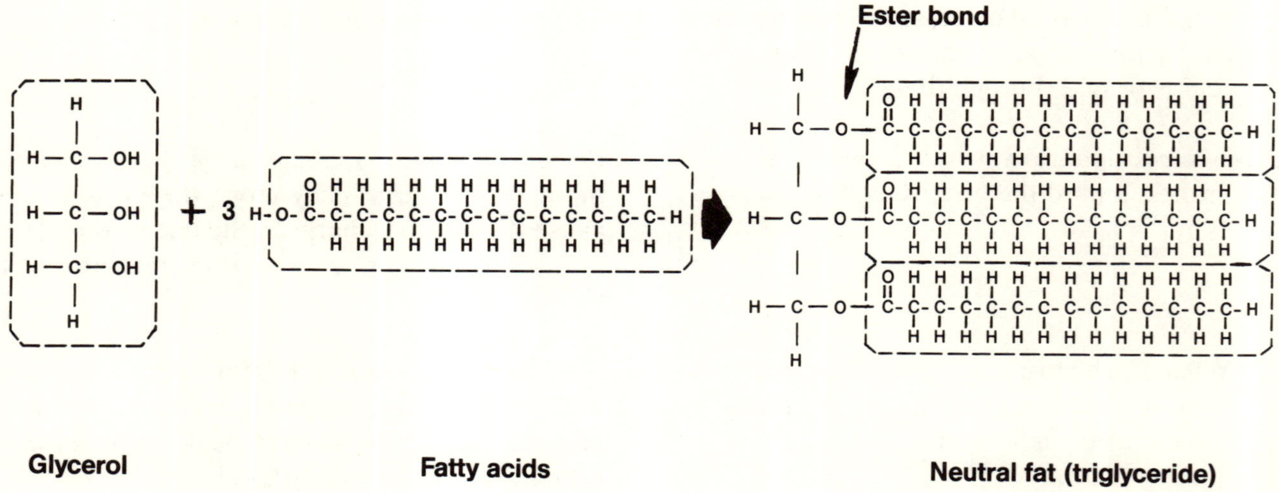

Figure 6–1. Formation of neutral fat (triglyceride).

Figure 6–2. The phosphate-containing end of the phospholipid is very polar and thus very soluble in water, whereas the long nonpolar fatty acid chains are very insoluble in water. The property of having one polar end (water soluble or **hydrophilic**) and one nonpolar end (water insoluble or **hydrophobic**) makes the phospholipids uniquely suitable to form the surrounding envelopes—**membranes**—of cells. Phospholipids are organized to form a phospholipid bilayer with the phospholipid polar (hydrophilic) ends projecting toward the water outside the cell *and* the water inside the cell (Figure 6–3). The nonpolar (hydrophobic) ends of the phospholipids face one another. Thus, cell membranes of the body are predominantly composed of phospholipid bilayers. Certain protein and sugar molecules are also wedged between the phospholipid bilayer and act as "receptors" for molecular messages coming from outside of the cell. These molecules serve many other purposes as well.

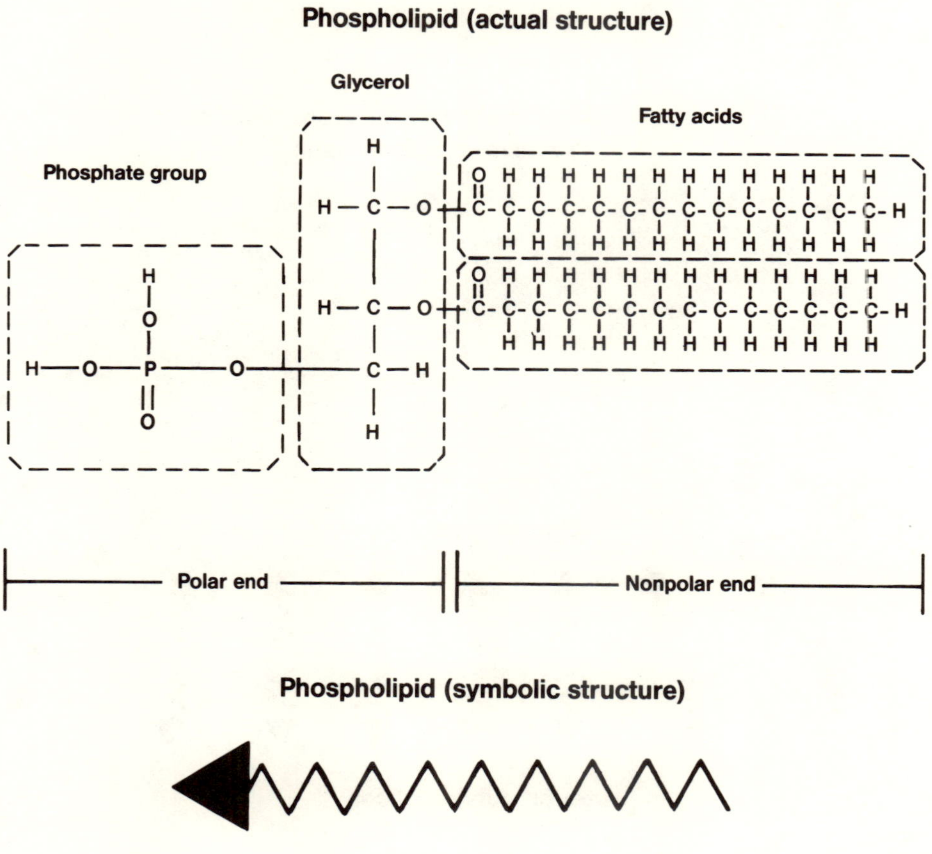

Figure 6–2. Actual and symbolic structure of the phospholipids.

The third class of lipids are the **steroids**. Steroids are structurally quite different from the neutral lipids and the phospholipids, but also are very insoluble in water. All steroid molecules are composed of a single five-sided carbon ring joined to three six-sided carbon rings (see Figure 6–4). Beneath the general steroid ring structure are shown three specific examples of steroids found in the human body: 1) **testosterone**, 2) **estrogen**, and 3) **cortisone (corticosteroids)**. As Figure 6–4 demonstrates, small changes in the steroid side-chain structure (denoted by arrows) can create steroid molecules with completely different biological activities. *Testosterone* is the principal male hormone in humans. *Estrogen* is the principal female hormone in humans. *Cortisone* is a hormone that produces many effects on body metabolism to allow an individual to react to stress. All three hormones are known to have different effects on immune system function.

Suggested Reading

Fasman, G. D. (ed.). *Handbook of Biochemistry and Molecular Biology*. Boca Raton, FL: CRC Press, 1976.

Lehninger, A. L. *Principles of Biochemistry*, 8th ed. New York: Worth, 1982.

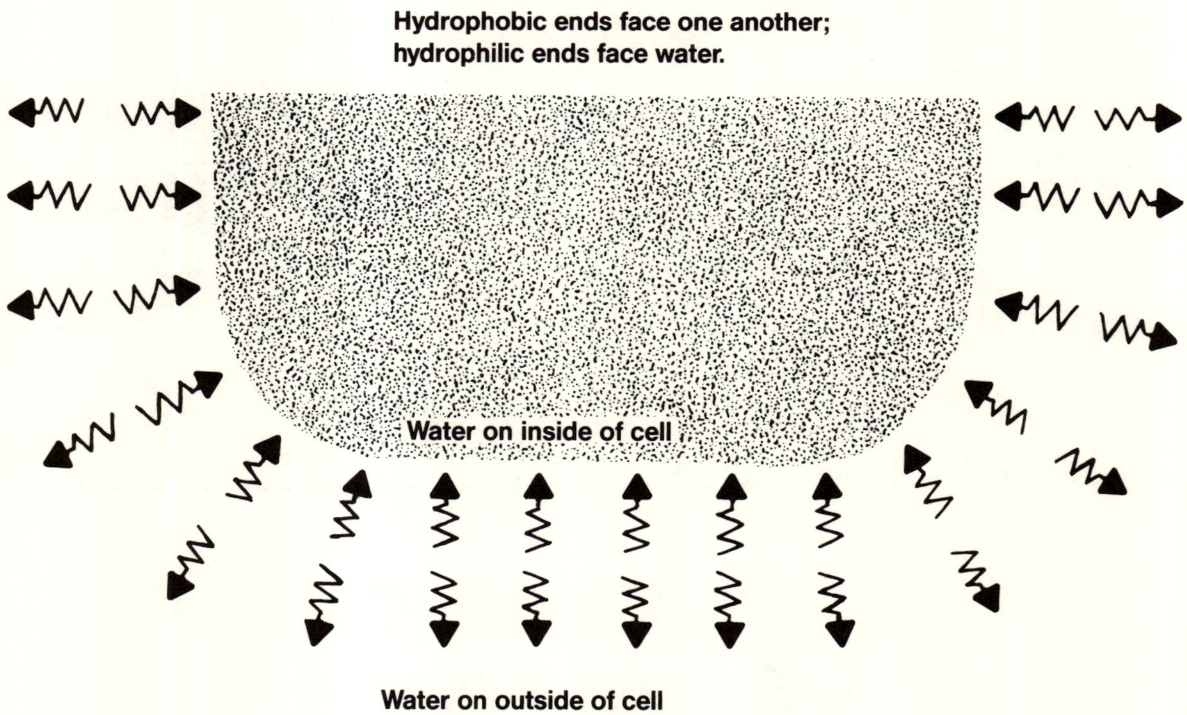

Figure 6–3. Organization of a phospholipid bilayer.

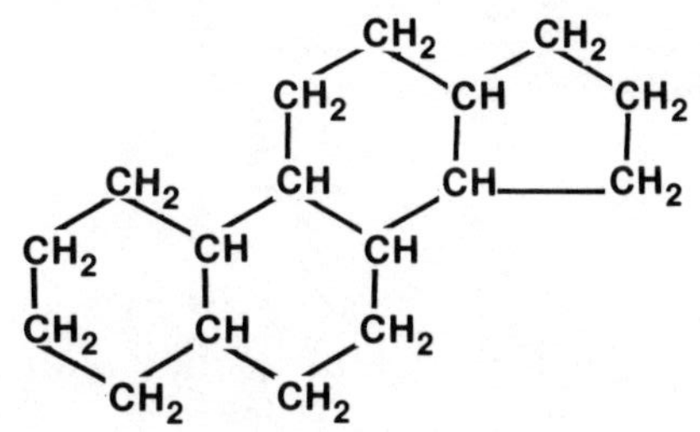

Basic steroid configuration

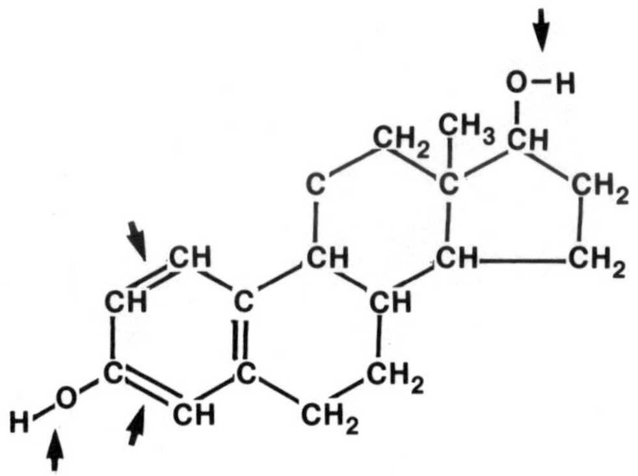

Estrogen

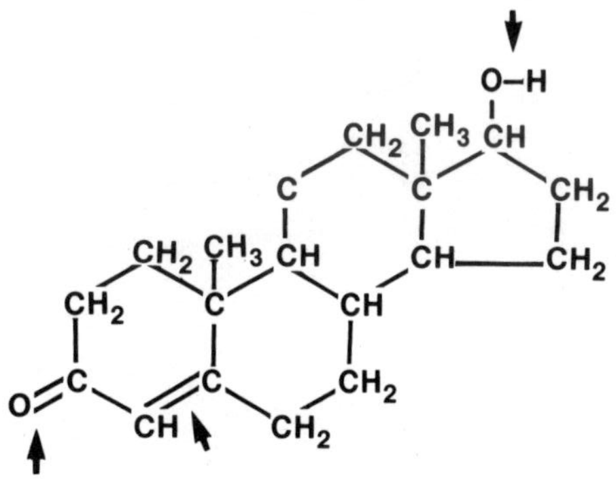

Testosterone

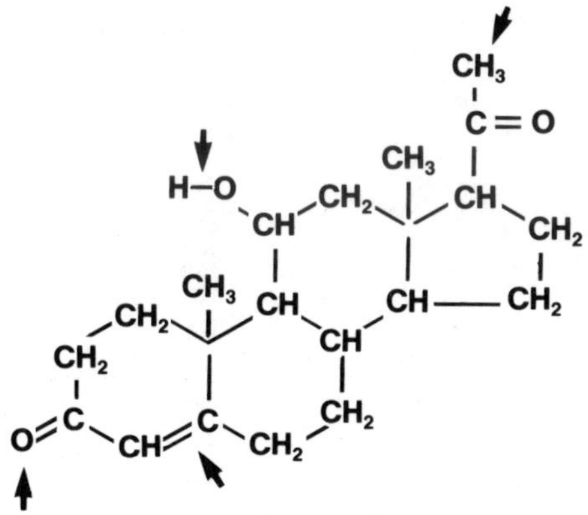

Cortisone

Figure 6–4. Basic steroid configuration with three representative examples.

REVIEW QUESTIONS for Lipids

1. What are lipids?

Lipids are a class of biomolecules that are relatively insoluble in water. This physical property is the basis for defining certain biomolecules as lipids. [p. 38]

2. Name the three major subclasses of lipids.

The three subclasses of lipids are neutral fats (triglycerides), phospholipids, and steroids. [p. 38]

3. Draw the general molecular structure of neutral fats (triglycerides).

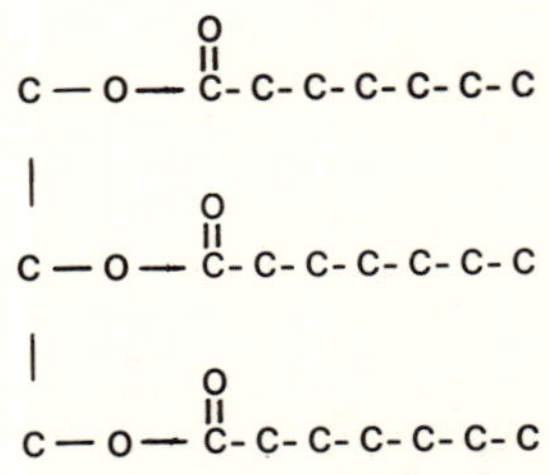

(Hydrogens are not drawn in.) [p. 38]

4. What are the component parts of each triglyceride molecule?

Triglyceride molecules have three fatty acids joined to a glycerol backbone by ester bonds. [p. 38]

5. Why are lipids relatively insoluble in water?

Lipid molecules contain very few polar or ionic groups within their structure. Thus, they are less likely to combine with water. They are mainly composed of carbon and hydrogen bonds (nonpolar covalent). [p. 39]

6. Draw the general molecular structure of phospholipids.

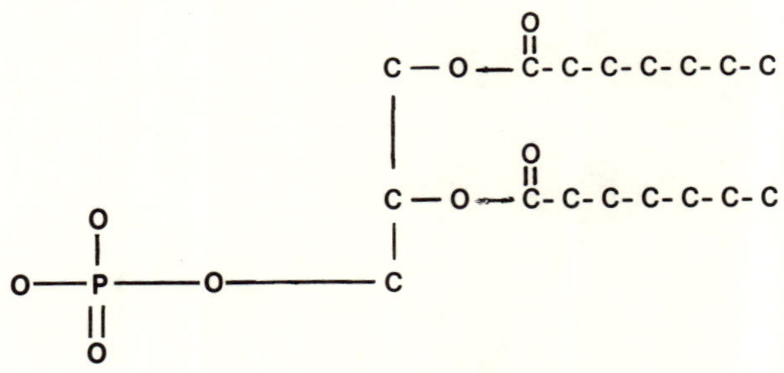

(Hydrogens are not drawn in.) [p. 39]

7. Why are phospholipids the principal component of cell membranes?

Phospholipids have a hydrophilic end which is soluble in water (both inside and outside the cell) and a hydrophobic end which will not mix with water. These properties cause phospholipids to form phospholipid bilayers. [p. 39]

8. Draw a phospholipid bilayer.

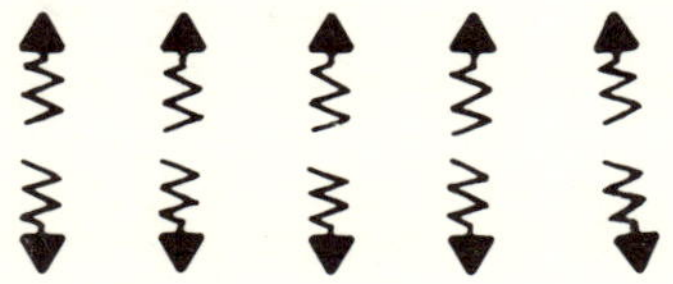

[p. 40]

9. Draw the general molecular structure of steroids.

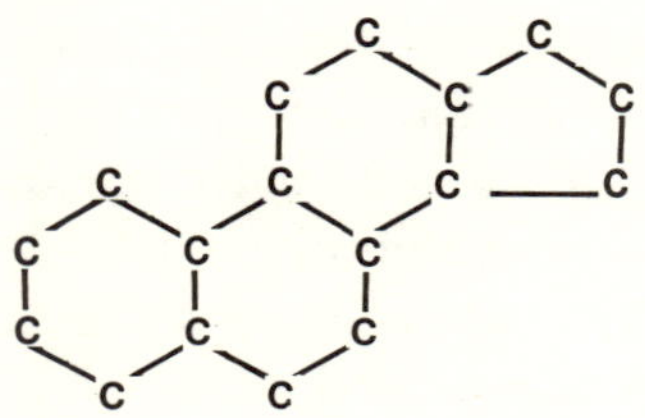

(Hydrogens are not drawn in.) [p.40–41]

CHAPTER 7

CARBOHYDRATES: MONOSACCHARIDES AND POLYSACCHARIDES

Carbohydrates (polysaccharides) play a critical role in the chemistry of the body because the chemical breakdown of carbohydrate molecules provides most of the chemical energy utilized by cells. (The breakdown of fats is a "backup" means of obtaining chemical energy.) Polysaccharides are composed of subunits called **monosaccharides** or sugars; two representative types are shown in Figure 7–1. One type of monosaccharide is **hexose**, which is shown as a six-sided carbon ring with an oxygen forming the upper right corner. There is, however, a total of six carbons in the entire molecule because a single carbon side-chain also exists at the top of the molecule. There are several different types of hexoses; the most important one is **glucose** (shown in Figure 7–1). Several five-sided sugars are known as **pentoses**; the example in Figure 7–1 is **ribose**. Pentose sugars have only five carbons; oxygen forms the uppermost corner of the ring structure and a single-carbon side-chain is attached. Simple sugars or monosaccharides can link together to form *polysaccharides*, also called *carbohydrates* (CHO), by the formation of a **glycosidic bond**. The process of having two or more sugars linked together by a glycosidic bond to form a polysaccharide is analogous to the process of having two or more separate amino acids joined together by a peptide bond to form a polypeptide. The precise reaction that generates the glycosidic bond is shown in Figure 7–2.

The first carbon to the right of the oxygen molecule in the first glucose ring moves close to the carbon on the opposite side of the oxygen in the second glucose ring. Hydrogen is removed from the –OH group on one carbon and the

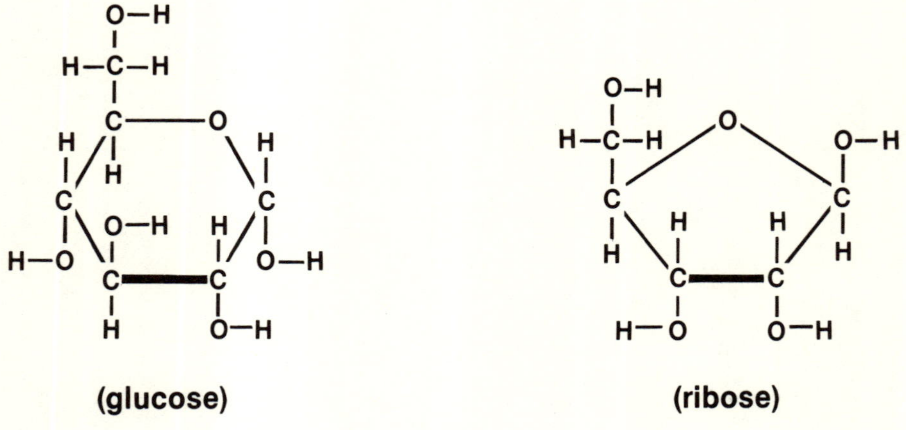

Figure 7–1. Representative structures of hexose (left) and pentose (right).

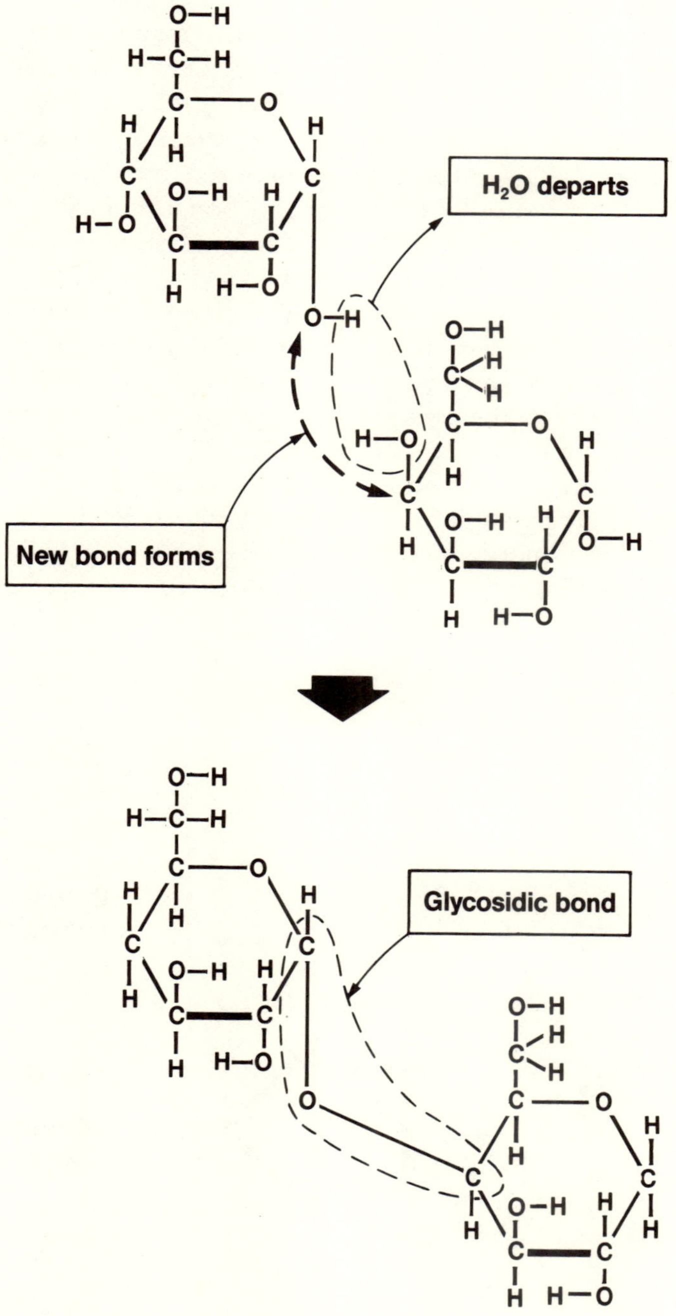

Figure 7–2. Glycosidic bond formation between two glucose molecules.

entire –OH group is removed from the carbon of the second glucose molecule. As a result, water is released and a nonpolar covalent bond (a shared electron pair that will not break apart in water) is formed between the oxygen attached to the carbon of one sugar molecule and the carbon of the second sugar molecule (the glycosidic bond). This reaction may continue with the sequential addition of other glucose (or other monosaccharide) molecules all linked by glycosidic bonds. Thus, the backbone of the polysaccharide is the repeating –sugar ring–O–sugar ring–O–sugar ring–O– bonds; the ring-like sugar structures extend like flags off of this backbone. Cells control the rate at which they synthesize specific polysaccharides by utilizing specific enzymes that promote glycosidic bond formation.

It is important to understand how sugars and starches are used as energy sources by the cells of the body. These biomolecules are high-energy molecules usually produced by plants. Animals (including humans) consume the high-energy molecules in order to extract the energy contained in their bonds. In the cells of our body, we possess enzymes that allow us to break down the bonds that hold sugars and starches together to release their stored energy. The specific reaction is shown in Figure 7–3. One molecule of glucose will react with six molecules of oxygen (O_2) to produce six molecules of carbon dioxide (CO_2) and six molecules of water (H_2O). The reason this reaction must take place in every cell of your body is because of an additional byproduct of the reaction—**energy**. The energy that is released when glucose molecules are catabolized (broken down) comes from the high-energy bonds present in the glucose molecule.

The catabolism of glucose by the cells of the body is analogous to the simple burning of wood. A high energy source (wood) reacts with oxygen (O_2) and, as a result, CO_2, H_2O, and energy (HEAT!) are produced. To regenerate a high energy molecule once again (such as glucose or wood), CO_2, H_2O, and added energy are required. This is exactly what plants do during **photosynthesis**. Plants take carbon dioxide (CO_2) from the air, water (H_2O) from the ground, and energy in the form of sunlight to create the

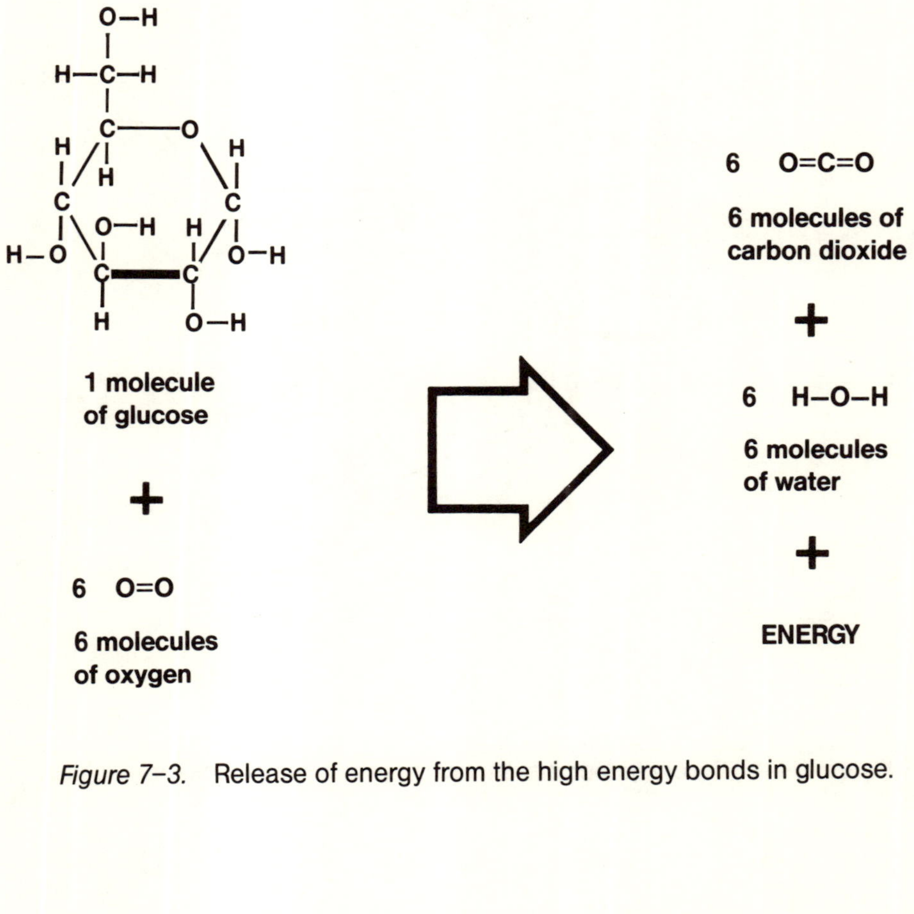

Figure 7–3. Release of energy from the high energy bonds in glucose.

wood we burn in our fireplaces and the sugar that we ingest as our principal cellular energy source. Remember that the catabolism of glucose by each cell is very similar to the burning of wood as a high energy source. In cells, however, the energy is not only released as heat but also is used internally to operate the various components of cell metabolism (to be reviewed in Chapter 9).

Monosaccharides and polysaccharides serve other functions beside providing energy for cell metabolism. When certain carbohydrates are inserted into the phospholipid bilayer of the cell membrane, they may act as receptors for incoming messages from outside the cell. Also, certain sugars may be released as signals to alter the function of other cells. In addition, certain polysaccharides may associate with proteins to protect them from degradation or to alter their function.

Suggested Reading

Davidson, E. A. *Carbohydrate Chemistry*. New York: Holt, Rinehart, & Winston, 1967.

Lehninger, A. L. *Principles of Biochemistry*, 8th ed. New York: Worth, 1982.

REVIEW QUESTIONS for Carbohydrates: Monosaccharides and Polysaccharides

1. What are the building blocks of polysaccharides (carbohydrates [CHO])?

Monosaccharides (single sugar molecules) are linked by chemical bonds called glycosidic bonds to form polysaccharides. [p. 44]

2. Name a representative hexose. Name a representative pentose.

Glucose
Ribose [p. 44]

3. Draw a structure of a hexose and of a pentose.

Hexose (glucose)

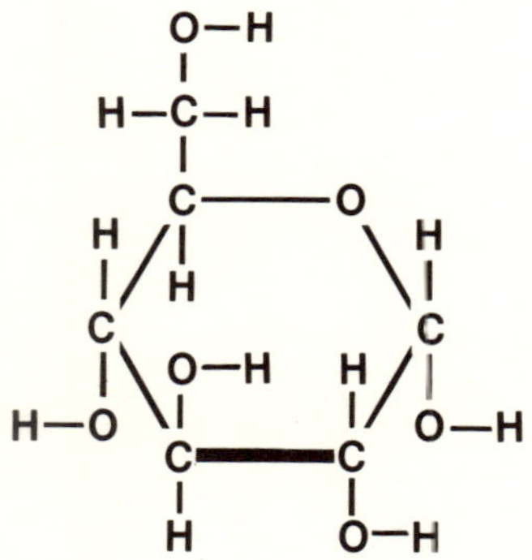

Pentose (ribose)

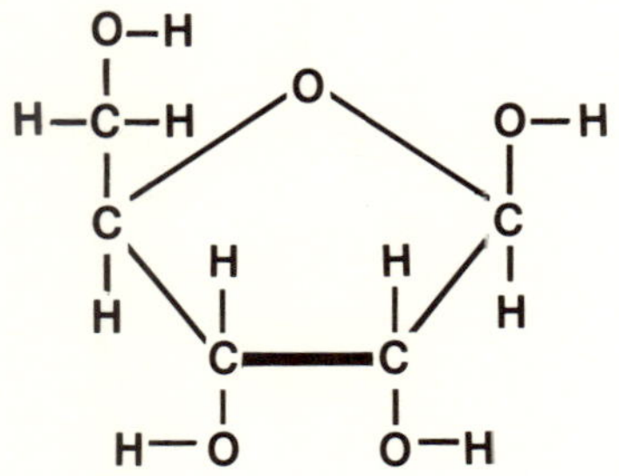

[p. 44]

4. Why do cells depend on sugars and starches to stay alive?

These molecules have high-energy bonds that are broken down to provide the needed energy to operate the metabolic processes of the cell. [p. 46]

5. Draw the reaction that allows cells to extract energy from the high energy molecule glucose.

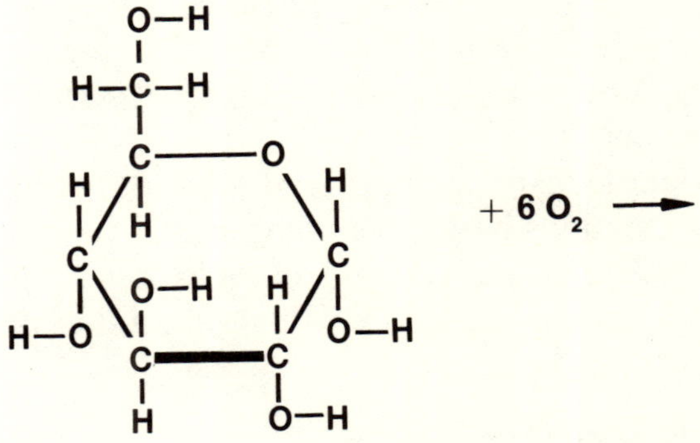

6 molecules of CO_2 +
6 molecules of H_2O + ENERGY
[p. 46]

CHAPTER 8

DNA AND RNA

We have previously reviewed three of the four major classes of biological molecules within the body: proteins, lipids, and carbohydrates. The fourth class, the **nucleic acids**, comprise a very small total of human body weight compared to the other classes. Nucleic acids are the largest and the most specialized molecules in the body. These molecules are of two types: **d**eoxyribo**n**ucleic **a**cid (**DNA**) and **r**ibo**n**ucleic **a**cid (**RNA**). RNA and DNA function in the storage and transfer of genetic information. They are the command center involved in the intricate genetic machinery of each cell. An organism's DNA determines what it is and what it can pass to its offspring (genetics). It is important to review and understand the biochemistry of DNA and RNA.

Both DNA and RNA are comprised of special molecules called **nucleic acid bases**. These special molecules are analogous to amino acids in proteins or monosaccharides in polysaccharides. There are two types of nucleic acid bases: the **purines** and the **pyrimidines**. As shown in Figure 8–1, the six-sided, ringed structure of the *purine* molecules is composed mainly of nitrogen, carbon, hydrogen, and oxygen. A five-sided ring structure is attached to one side of the six-sided ring. There are two purines, **adenine** (A) and **guanine** (G). The **pyrimidines** are structurally similar to the *purines*. The *pyrimidines* have a single, six-sided molecule composed of the same elements as the purines, but have no five-sided ring. The pyrimidines are **cytosine** (C) and **thymine** (T). It is important to note that in RNA, *thymine* (T) is replaced by a slightly different pyrimidine, **uracil** (U). To be used as the building blocks of DNA and RNA, nucleic acid bases must be assembled with specific sugars and phosphate groups to create essential subunits known as **nucleotides** (reviewed below).

Molecular Structure of DNA

DNA molecules are principally found in the center of each cell in a structure known as the **cell nucleus** (to be reviewed in Chapter 9). The structure of DNA is very similar to that of polypeptides. Like polypeptides, the DNA molecule has a backbone that forms a straight chain. As shown in Figure 8–2, this backbone is made up of molecules of the sugar (S) **deoxyribose** which are held together by **special phosphate bonds** (P) (*not* glycosidic bonds). Attached to each sugar is one of the four different types of nucleic acid bases—A, T, G, or C. Thus, the DNA molecule is composed of linear chains of sugar (S)–phosphate (P)–nucleic acid base (A, T, G or C) **complexes**, which are called *nucleotides*. DNA is often schematically represented as a ladder-type configuration that has been slightly twisted. This twisted ladder conformation is called a *double helix* and is shown in Figure 8–3. Notice that the sugars (S) connect via the phosphate (P) polar covalent bonds to form the side rails of the ladder. The rungs of the twisted ladder are created by the nucleic acid bases that are attached to a sugar (S) on each side. Each nucleic acid faces an opposing nucleic acid within each rung. The opposing nucleic acid bases are specifically paired to each other by electrical attractions, represented by ---- in Figure 8–3. The pairing of nucleic acid bases in each rung of the DNA ladder is very specific. If one side of the ladder rung has a *purine*, the opposite side must have a *pyrimidine* facing the purine. There is always one purine and one pyrimidine paired together to form each rung of the DNA twisted ladder. They cannot be assembled in any other fashion: two pyrimidines will not electrically attract one another to allow a maintained con-

PURINES

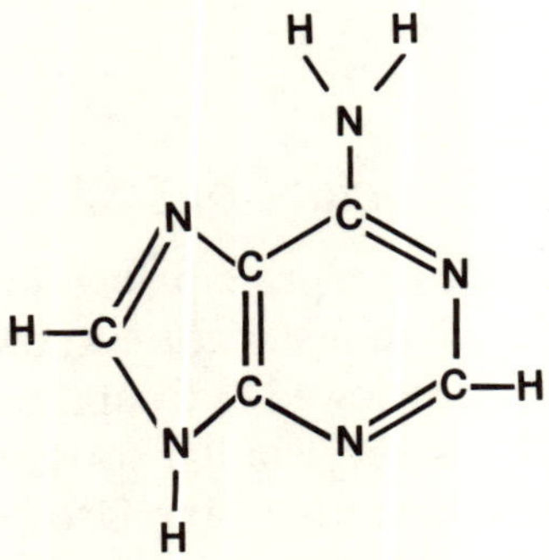

Adenine (A)

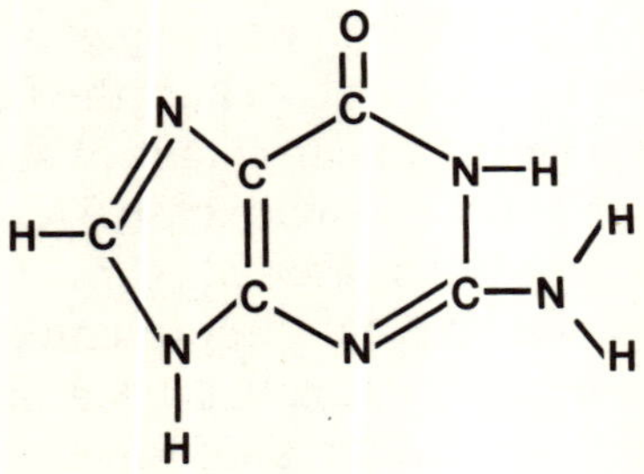

Guanine (G)

PYRIMIDINES

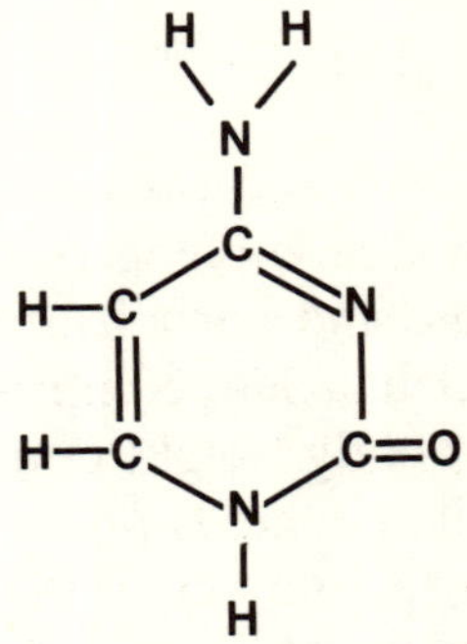

Cytosine (C)

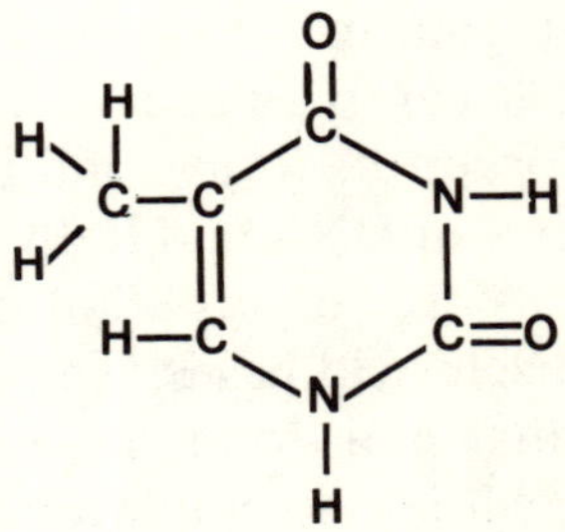

Thymine (T)

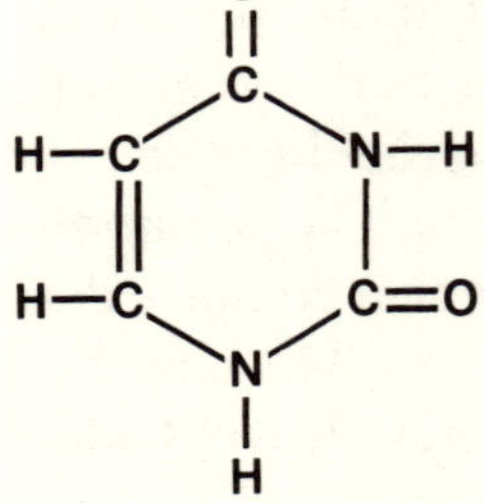

Uracil (U)-(replaces thymine in RNA)

Figure 8–1. The five types of nucleic acid bases found in RNA and DNA.

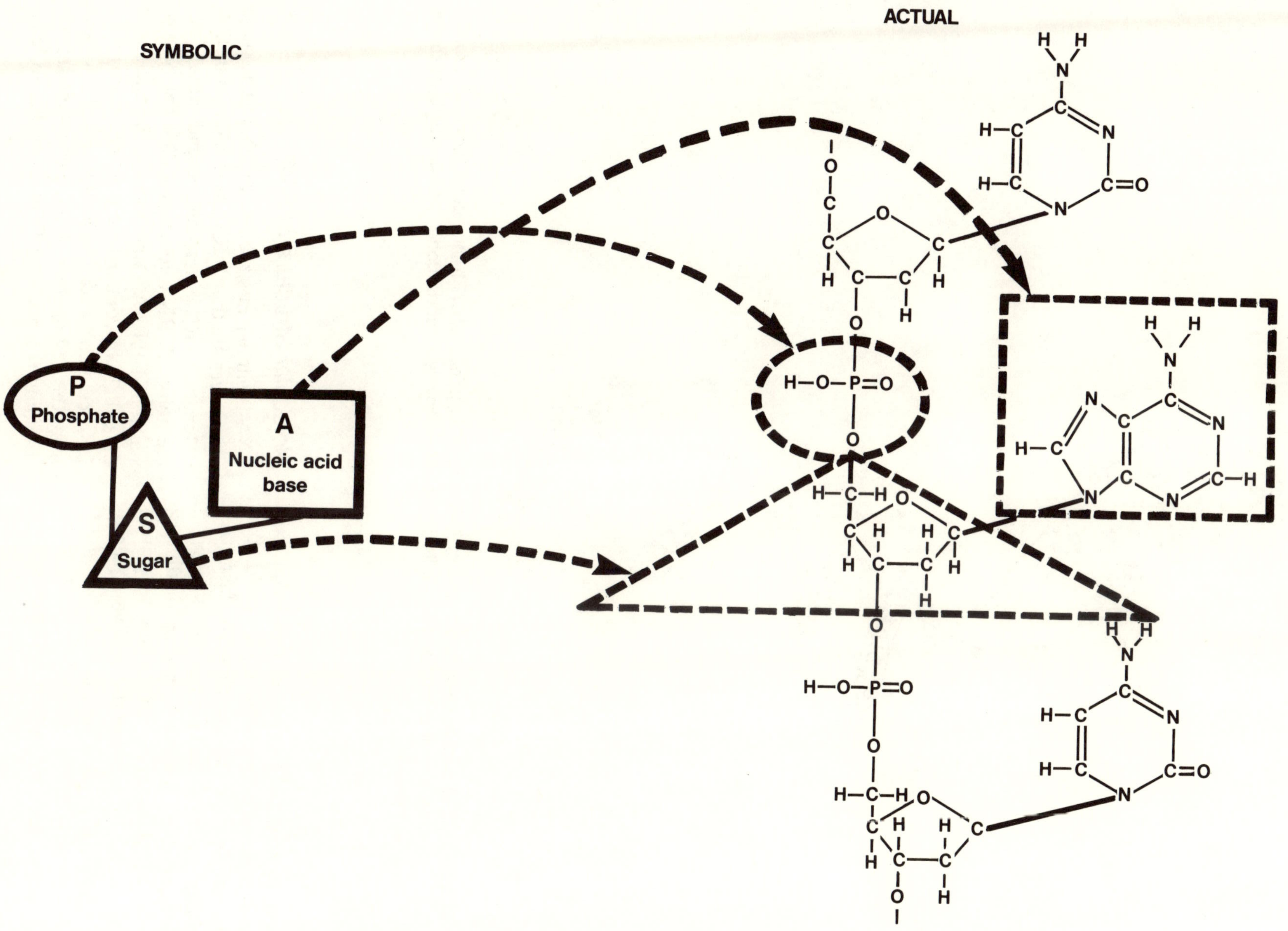

Figure 8–2. Representation of the components of a DNA chain.

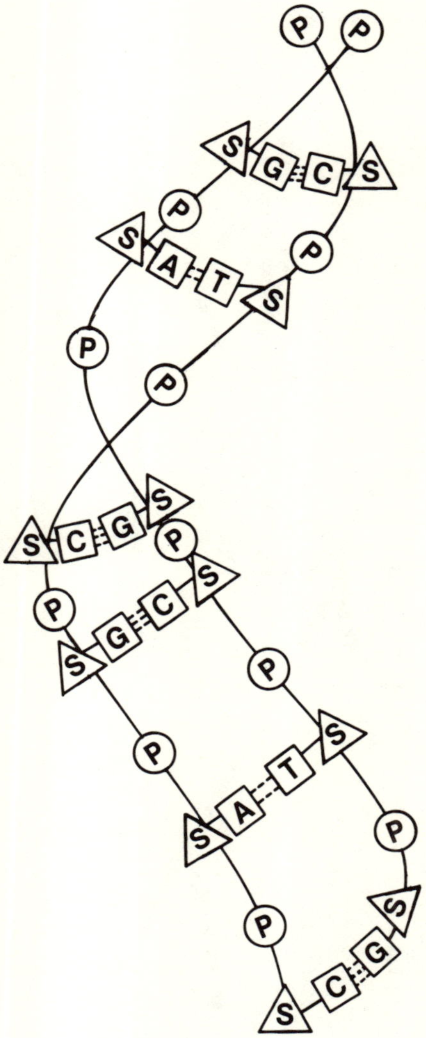

Figure 8–3. The DNA double helix. Two chains of DNA (sugar [S], phosphate [P], and nucleic acid [A,T,G, or C] groups) form the double helix. (Solid lines indicate covalent bonds; dotted lines indicate electrical attractions.)

nection. In contrast, two purine molecules, because of their extra five-sided rings, would take up too much room in the rung. In fact, the matching of purines and pyrimidines is specific to the point that each purine and pyrimidine is exactly paired. Adenine (A) is always paired with thymine (T); guanine (G) is always paired with cytosine (C). Electrostatic attractions (not covalent bonds) are the basis for this specific attraction between the nucleic acid bases in the DNA molecule.

Molecular Structure of RNA

RNA is similar in structure to DNA. The main differences are that 1) RNA is smaller than DNA in length, 2) RNA is a single strand (not a double helix), 3) RNA contains a different type of sugar, and 4) RNA is able to leave the nucleus of the cell. RNA contains the pentose sugar *ribose*; DNA contains *deoxyribose*. RNA is able to travel from the cell nucleus to the cell **cytoplasm** surrounding the nucleus; DNA is unable to leave the nucleus. DNA is the site where the genetic code for protein assembly is maintained; RNA *copies* the genetic information from the DNA molecule and transports it to the **ribosome**, the protein-synthesizing **organelle** (a cellular structure) found in the cell cytoplasm. Proteins needed by the cell are synthesized in the ribosome.

Three types of RNA function in the **transcription** (copy) and **translation** (decoding) of DNA so that proteins are made. Three RNA forms are: 1) **messenger RNA** (mRNA), 2) **transfer RNA** (tRNA), and 3) **ribosomal RNA** (rRNA). Their functions are extremely complex but their main differences are not: *mRNA* copies the DNA strands and then passes the genetic code from the nucleus to the ribosomes in the cytoplasm; *tRNA* is involved in selecting various single amino acids from the cytoplasm as they are required during the assembly of polypeptides by the ribosome; and *rRNA* is actually the structural backbone of the ribosome.

DNA Segments Copied into mRNA Strands

After the basic structure of DNA and RNA is understood, consider the mechanics of how information stored within DNA is transferred (transcribed) into RNA. Remember that DNA contains all of the genetic information of an organism. More specifically, the genetic information contains codes for the synthesis of the proteins needed to operate the cell.

Each side rail of the DNA twisted ladder is held together with strong sugar–phosphate (S–P) covalent bonds that are not easily broken. However, the nucleic acid base pairs forming the rungs of the twisted ladder are held together by electrical attractions that will break much more readily than the S–P bond. This allows the DNA strand to unwind (unzip) from its double helix form into its two separate strands so that an exact messenger RNA mirror image can be copied (transcribed) from the message-containing DNA strand. This process of DNA unzipping and mRNA transcription is shown in Figure 8–4. The transcribed mRNA then travels through the nuclear membrane to the cytoplasm, where it is decoded (translated) by the ribosome.

For the sake of simplicity, picture the ribosome as a structure constructed mainly of rRNA, with two tubes running through it, as shown in Figure 8–5. It manufactures proteins by reading the code found on mRNA molecules much as a ticker-tape machine reads punched tape. The code on each mRNA strand tells the ribosome which protein to synthesize. It is known as a **triplet code** because the code that has been transcribed from the DNA onto the mRNA molecule is read (translated) in *groups of three nucleotides* by the ribosome. Since there are four nucleic acid bases in the mRNA molecule (A, G, C, U) and each mRNA strand is decoded (translated) in groups of three bases, there are 64 different triplet codes that can be read by the ribosome ($4 \times 4 \times 4 = 64$). Each triplet code tells the ribosome additional information about the protein being assembled. Some triplet codes instruct the ribosome to add specific amino acids, while others tell the ribosome to start or to stop the assembly of a given protein. Because there are 20 common amino acids and there are 64 combinations of triplet codes, there is obviously some redundancy in the *triplet coding system*. Several different triplet codes might request the same amino acid or may be read as a stop or start signal. As shown in Figure 8–5, the ribosome takes the mRNA into its upper tube and *translates* each triplet code to determine the specific single amino acids required for the assembly of the desired protein. Single amino acids are carried from the cytoplasm to the ribosome by tRNA (not shown in Figure 8–5). The required amino acids are fed into the bottom tube and are strung together by the formation of peptide bonds between them. The desired polypeptide protein exits from the bottom tube and the decoded mRNA is discarded from the top tubes. The translated mRNA may then be processed by another ribosome if further protein synthesis is required.

Suggested Reading

Davidson, J. N. *The Biochemistry of the Nucleic Acids*. New York: Academic Press, 1972.

Lehninger, A. L. *Principles of Biochemistry*, 8th ed. New York: Worth, 1982.

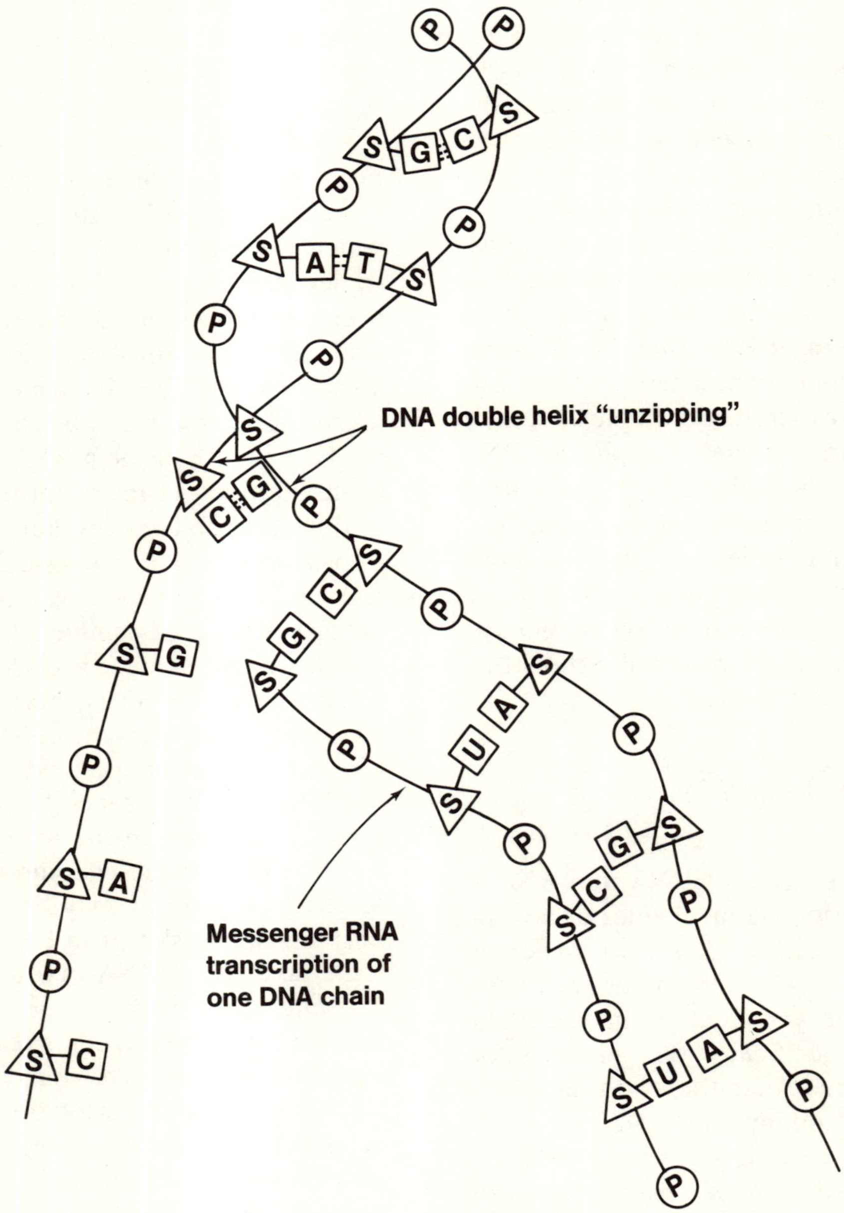

Figure 8–4. The transcription of a DNA chain.

REVIEW QUESTIONS for DNA and RNA

1. What class of biomolecules do RNA and DNA belong to?

RNA and DNA belong to the class of nucleic acids. [p. 49]

2. What are the building blocks of DNA and RNA?

The building blocks of DNA and RNA are specialized molecules called nucleic acid bases. Nucleic acid bases become complexed to specific sugars and phosphate groups to form nucleotides. [p. 49]

1. **mRNA enters ribosome (top tube); free amino acids (a.a.) await.**

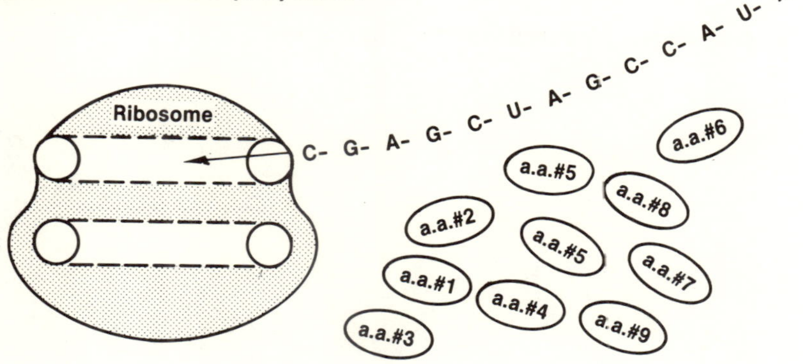

2. **mRNA triplet code is translated: specific amino acids, as directed by the triplet code, enter bottom tube and peptide bonds are formed.**

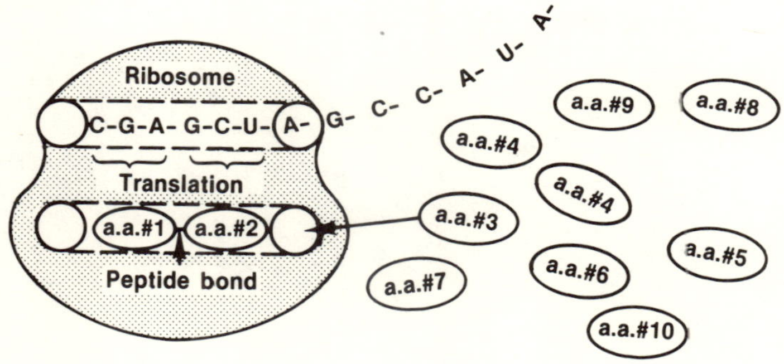

3. **Translated mRNA exits top tube; protein exits bottom tube.**

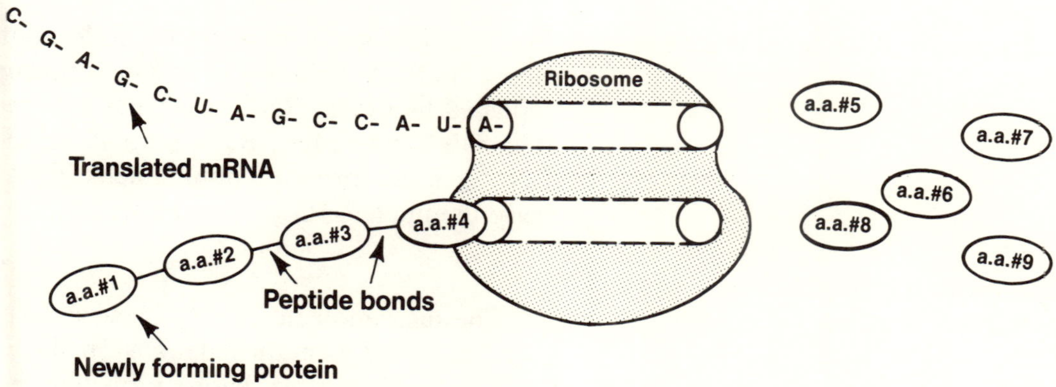

Figure 8–5. Formation of a peptide by a ribosome.

3. What are the two major types of nucleic acid bases?

The two types of nucleic acid bases are the purines and the pyrimidines. [p. 49]

4. Draw a purine structure. Name the purines.

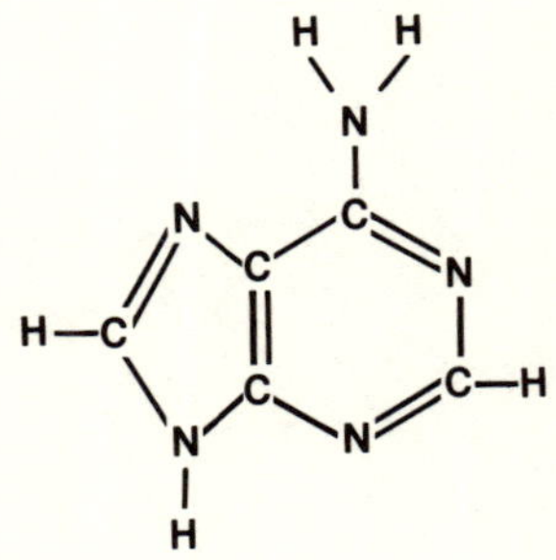

Adenine

Adenine (A) and guanine (G) are the purines. [p. 49–50]

5. Draw a pyrimidine. Name the pyrimidines.

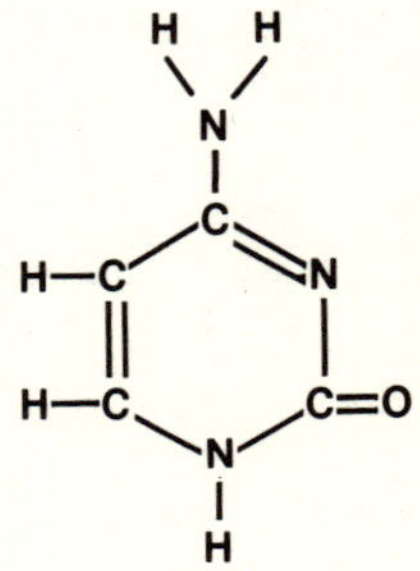

Cytosine

Thymine (T), cytosine (C), and uracil (U) are the pyrimidines. [p. 49–50]

6. What are the major differences between DNA and RNA?

In DNA the sugar is deoxyribose; RNA contains ribose. In RNA, the nucleic acid base thymine is replaced by uracil. RNA molecules are smaller than DNA molecules. RNA is single-stranded; DNA is in the form of a double helix. RNA can leave the nucleus; DNA cannot. [p. 52]

7. Compare DNA with a twisted ladder.
   A) What molecules form the side rails?
   B) What molecules form the rungs?
   C) How are the nucleic acid bases of one DNA chain bound to the opposing nucleic acid bases of the other chain?

A) The sugar molecule deoxyribose and a phosphate bond form the side rails. [p. 49]
B) The nucleic acid bases form the rungs. [p. 49]
C) Electrical attractions hold the nucleic acid bases together. [p. 49]

D) Why can a purine only match with a pyrimidine in the DNA chain?

D) Purines and pyrimidines are the only molecules that take up the exact amount of space allowed for the rungs within the DNA molecule and also have the proper required electrical attractions. [p. 49–52]

E) Why does adenine (A) only link with thymine (T) and guanine (G) only link with cytosine (C)?

E) The electrical attractions are only found at the right places in the A–T or the G–C combination. [p. 52]

8. What does DNA code for?

DNA codes for proteins. [p. 53]

9. Name the three types of RNA and describe their functions.

1) Messenger RNA (mRNA) copies the DNA strand and transfers the genetic code from the nucleus to the ribosome.
2) Ribosomal RNA (rRNA) makes up the ribosome structure.
3) Transfer RNA (tRNA) brings free amino acids into the ribosome as required for protein assembly. [p. 53]

10. What organelle is the site of protein synthesis?

The ribosome is the site of protein synthesis. [p. 53]

11. How does the DNA code reach the ribosome?

The DNA code sequence is copied onto mRNA (transcription), which is capable of migrating to the ribosome. [p. 53]

12. In what specific form is the DNA code given?

The code is given as a triplet code: three nucleic acid bases in sequence code for one message, usually a specific amino acid. [p. 53]

13. How many total types of messages can exist in the triplet code?

A total of 64 total triplet codes are available for protein synthesis. These messages code for the assembly of 20 amino acids into any given polypeptide. The triplet code is somewhat redundant. [p. 53]

14. The ribosome can be visualized as a structure with two tubes running through it.

A) What function occurs in the top tube?

A) The decoding (translation) of mRNA occurs in the top tube. [p. 53, 55]

B) What function occurs in the bottom tube?

B) The construction of proteins from various free amino acids occurs in the bottom tube (formation of peptide bonds to create a new polypeptide). [p. 53, 55]

PART II

CELL BIOLOGY AND GENETICS

After developing an understanding of the principal biomolecules and certain of their functions, try now to visualize these biomolecules as they come together at the level of the *cell*. The cell is the basic life form for all organisms. Human beings are multicellular organisms in which each cell cooperates for the mutual benefit of all cells. In the following chapters, the function of each type of biomolecule within each cell is demonstrated. The details on how each cell survives in the complicated environment that exists inside the human body is presented. Finally, *how* the genetic information stored inside the nucleus of each cell is passed on to other cells, and how the genetic information stored in the nucleus of each cell affects the function of that cell is reviewed. With this information in hand, the reader will be prepared to understand the detailed functioning of a specific group of cells in the body: the human immune system.

CHAPTER 9

CELLS: ORGANIZATION AND FUNCTION

We have completed a review of the four principal biomolecules: 1) proteins, 2) lipids, 3) carbohydrates, and 4) RNA and DNA. These biomolecules come together in their most basic organized form at the level of the individual cells. The various cell types in the body tend to have different functions, but the general structure of most cells is the same.

As shown in Figure 9–1, cells possess an outer **cell membrane** that envelopes the entire cell. The cell membrane is made of a phospholipid bilayer (described in Chapter 6). Interspersed throughout the phospholipid bilayer are protein and carbohydrate receptors that allow the cell to receive incoming messages from the outside. The major structure inside the cell membrane is the **nucleus**. The nucleus consists of concentrated packets of DNA called **chromosomes**. Each chromosome consists of one very long twisted ladder molecule of DNA. Each human nucleus consists of 23 pairs of chromosomes, a total of 46 chromosomes per nucleus (reviewed in Chapter 10). The nucleus is bounded by a **nuclear membrane**. Everything inside the cell that is not within the nucleus is **cytoplasm**, which contains numerous structures. The most important cytoplasmic structures, or *organelles*, include 1) the **ribosomes**, 2) the **rough endoplasmic reticulum** (**RER**), 3) the **mitochondria**, 4) the **Golgi apparatus**, and 5) the **cytoskeleton**.

The *ribosomes* have been reviewed in Chapter 8. These cytoplasmic structures are protein-synthesizing factories that translate the messenger RNA that was transcribed from DNA, into the protein for which mRNA codes. In the *rough endoplasmic reticulum* the ribosomes congregate along a smooth receptacle that collects the proteins assembled by the ribosomes.

The *mitochondria* are energy factories. These organelles are responsible for supplying the energy needs of the rest of the cell. Mitochondria take molecules such as sugar and oxygen from the bloodstream and convert them into H_2O and CO_2, and release the energy stored in the bonds of the high energy fuel (reviewed in Chapter 7). This energy is transferred to a biomolecule known as **ATP** (*a*denosine *tri*phosphate). In the form of ATP, energy can be stored for later use by the cell for other metabolic processes.

The *Golgi apparatus* consists of little sacs in the cytoplasm. They collect secretory products, such as proteins from the ribosomes, that are destined to be transported to the outside of the cell. A cell has particular need of the Golgi apparatus if it is a secretory cell (secreting proteins outside its cell membrane to the rest of the body). The Golgi apparatus can be visualized as empty bags in the cytoplasm which fill up with secretory protein as it is being assembled by the ribosome. The Golgi apparatus then transports the contained secretory product to the cell membrane, where it is dumped on the outside of the cell.

The entire cell membrane envelope is supported by a tent or frame-like mechanism known as the *cytoskeleton*. The cytoskeleton consists of two types of fibers, **microtubules** and **microfilaments**, which emanate from a structure located in the center of the cell known as the **centriole**. The cytoskeleton not only supports the cell but also aids in moving the cell (locomotion) when necessary.

From a functional point of view, the cells to be studied in Parts III and IV of this book (the leukocytes) operate just like any individual organism. They interact with the outside environment, take

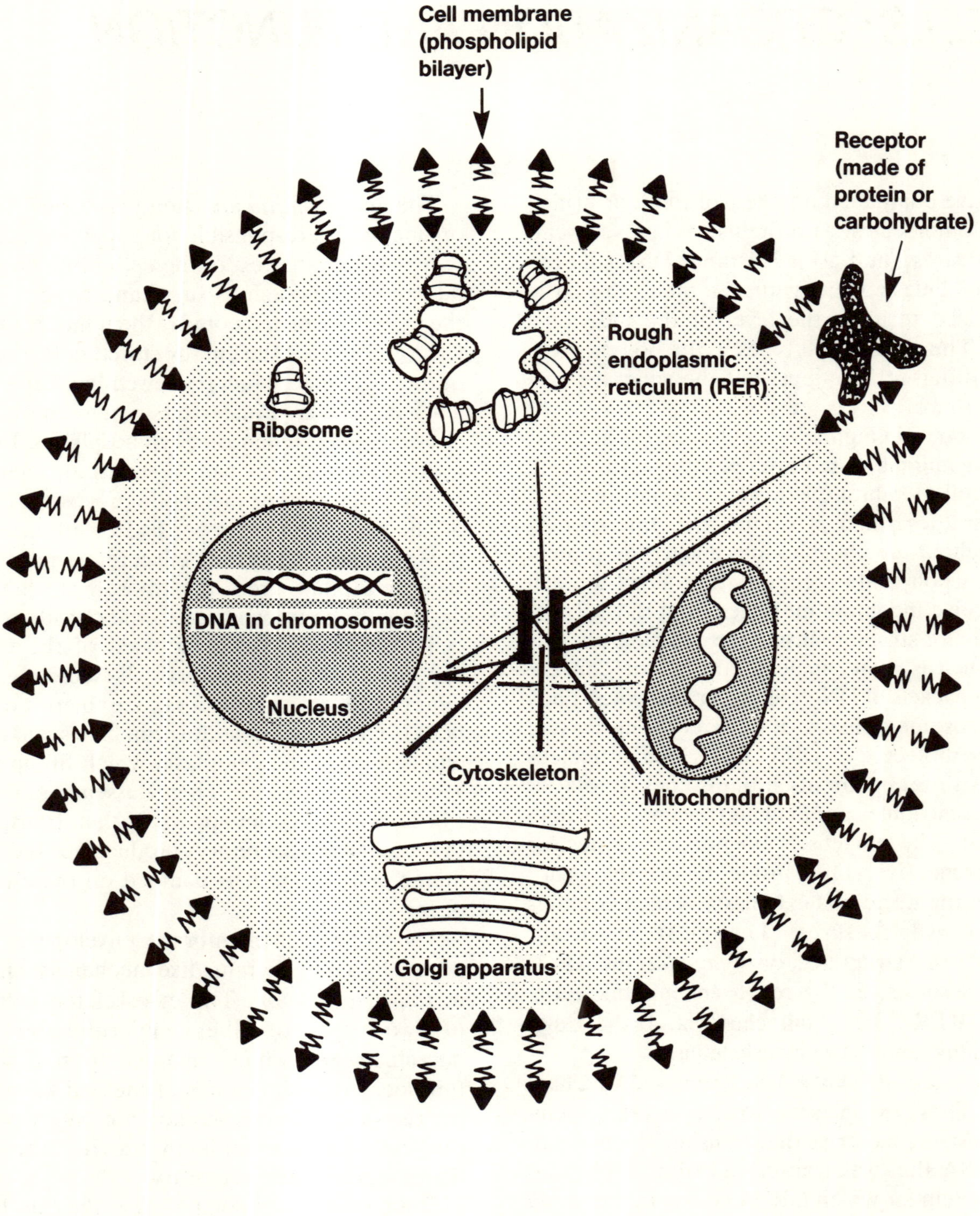

Figure 9–1. Examples of cellular organelles.

in nutrients, and expel waste products. All substances entering and leaving the cell must pass through the cell membrane, which is a phospholipid bilayer. The mitochondria absorb O_2 and molecules such as carbohydrates (CHO) from the environment and break down the CHO into H_2O, CO_2, and energy. The energy stored in the CHO bonds is harnessed by the mitochondria in high-energy ATP molecules available for the energy needs of the rest of the cell.

DNA is the controlling molecule of the cell. Housed in the nucleus, the DNA possesses the codes for all of the characteristics of the cell. The *DNA triplet code* instructs the ribosome on how to assemble every *protein* needed by the cell via mRNA molecules. Indirectly, the DNA also codes for all of the other biomolecules that a cell possesses, from lipids to carbohydrates to DNA and RNA synthesis. This is because DNA codes for the three basic types of proteins. Although a minority of all cellular proteins are *structural* or in the *other* category, most proteins are *enzymes*. The purpose of enzymes is to catalyze chemical reactions so they proceed much more quickly than they ordinarily would. The cell that expresses the DNA coding for any specific protein enzyme will be able to make the product of the reaction that the enzyme catalyzes. The cell that does not contain DNA, or does not synthesize the mRNA to make the enzyme, will not make that reaction product. Critical enzymes exist for lipid, polysaccharide, protein, DNA and RNA synthesis. Thus, all cell functions trace their origins back to the DNA code found in the cell nucleus and the protein products of that code.

Suggested Reading

Karp, G. *Cell Biology*. New York: McGraw-Hill, 1979.

Wolfe, S. L. *Biology of the Cell*. Belmont, CA: Wadsworth, 1981.

REVIEW QUESTIONS for Cells: Organization and Function

1. What is the basic composition of the cell membrane?

   The cell membrane is composed of a phospholipid bilayer and receptors. [p. 59]

2. What kind of molecules are found in the cell chromosomes?

   DNA molecules are organized in packets called chromosomes. [p. 59]

3. What are five organelles found in the cytoplasm?

   The ribosomes, the rough endoplasmic reticulum, the Golgi apparatus, the mitochondrion, and the cytoskeleton are found in the cytoplasm. [p. 59]

4. Where does protein assembly occur in the cell?

   Protein assembly occurs in the ribosome. [p. 59]

5. What organelle supplies the energy needs of the cell?

   The mitochondrion ("powerhouse of the cell") produces energy. [p. 59]

6. What is the overall chemical reaction that occurs in the mitochondrion to provide the energy for the cell?

   1 Glucose molecule + 6 molecules of $O_2 \rightarrow$ 6 molecules of CO_2 + 6 molecules of H_2O + Energy [p. 59]

7. What is the chemical form in which energy is stored in the cells?

Energy is stored in molecules of ATP (adenosine triphosphate) [p. 59]

8. What is the function of the Golgi apparatus?

The Golgi apparatus packages secretory cell products such as protein for transfer to the outside of the cell. [p. 59]

9. What is the rough endoplasmic reticulum?

The rough endoplasmic reticulum is a group of ribosomes clustered around a smooth collection sack. [p. 59]

10. What is the function of the cytoskeleton?

The cytoskeleton supports the cell membrane and aids in cell locomotion. [p. 59]

11. What types of proteins are made in the ribosome?

Structural, enzymatic, and "other" proteins are made in the ribosome. [p. 59]

12. What are enzymes?

Enzymes are special proteins that catalyze (promote) chemical reactions. [p. 61]

13. How does the DNA of a cell code for the lipids, carbohydrates, and nucleic acids that a cell synthesizes?

If a cell possesses the specific DNA that codes for the protein enzyme that catalyzes the synthesis of the lipid, carbohydrate, or nucleic acid, and if the DNA code is transcribed by mRNA, then that cell can produce the needed product. However, if the cell lacks that DNA code for the needed protein enzyme or if the mRNA does not transcribe the DNA code, no product can be made. [p. 61]

CHAPTER 10

HOW CELLS OF THE BODY SURVIVE

Although each living cell has a distinct type of function, the cells of the body must cooperate so that the entire organism can live. It is clear that the dominant cells in the body are the brain cells; without intact brain cells, the human is not technically alive. In contrast, the organism can lose the cells of one arm or both arms, and even noncritical internal organs, and still stay alive. Most of the cells of the body and most of the organ systems of the body exist to support the existence of the brain. Nevertheless, life at the level of the individual cell (such as the leukocytes of the immune system—Part III) is surprisingly the same most everywhere in the body.

As shown in Figure 10–1, most cells exist along a lifeline tube called a **capillary**. The capillaries are thin-walled tubes through which the **arterial blood** of the body must pass on the way to the **veins** before returning to the heart. The arterial blood has four major characteristics: 1) it is under high pressure, having recently been ejected from the heart; 2) it is high in nutrients such as glucose and amino acids; 3) it is high in the critical life-giving gas oxygen, which is needed for the metabolism of carbohydrates (as previously described); and 4) arterial blood has low osmotic vacuum (discussed below). However, none of the valuable properties of arterial blood are any good to the cells of the body because nothing can escape through the thick walls of the arteries to the cells. Instead, the arterial blood must enter the thin-walled capillaries. The capillary walls are permeable to small molecules such as amino acids and glucose and allow for the transport of oxygen to the cells of each tissue. High pressure exists at the arterial end of the capillaries. Under high pressure, glucose and amino acids pour out into tissue spaces known as **interstitial space** to nourish the cells. It is important to note that the capillaries are only semipermeable. For the most part, large proteins of the blood, such as albumin, and most blood cells remain inside the capillaries. As the fluid is forced out of the capillary at the arterial end, the capillary fluid becomes water depleted and the large albumin proteins become concentrated (a situation known as **osmotic vacuum**). As the fluid pressure inside the capillary drops (when the blood reaches the venous end of the capillary) and the osmotic vacuum rises, the nutrient-rich fluid that was pushed into the interstitial space to nourish the cells now returns into the capillary. However, the fluid returns with one important difference: The cells have absorbed the nutrients and added waste products such as carbon dioxide and urea (a major component of urine). These waste products enter the venous end of the capillary to flow into the veins. When blood returns to the thick-walled veins, no exchange of gases or nutrients can occur. The venous blood returns to the heart to be distributed to the lungs where CO_2 is removed and O_2 is infused, then travels to the kidneys where the urea and other waste products are filtered out. Most cells in the body, including the immune system cells, must be supplied with oxygen and nutrients by the capillary system. If any cells die and become degraded, the large molecules (proteins and DNA, for example) cannot enter the capillaries. These molecules do not stay trapped in the interstitial space; instead, they are drained toward the heart by a very low pressure drainage system known as the **lymphatics**. The immune system is intimately associated with the interstitial drainage system.

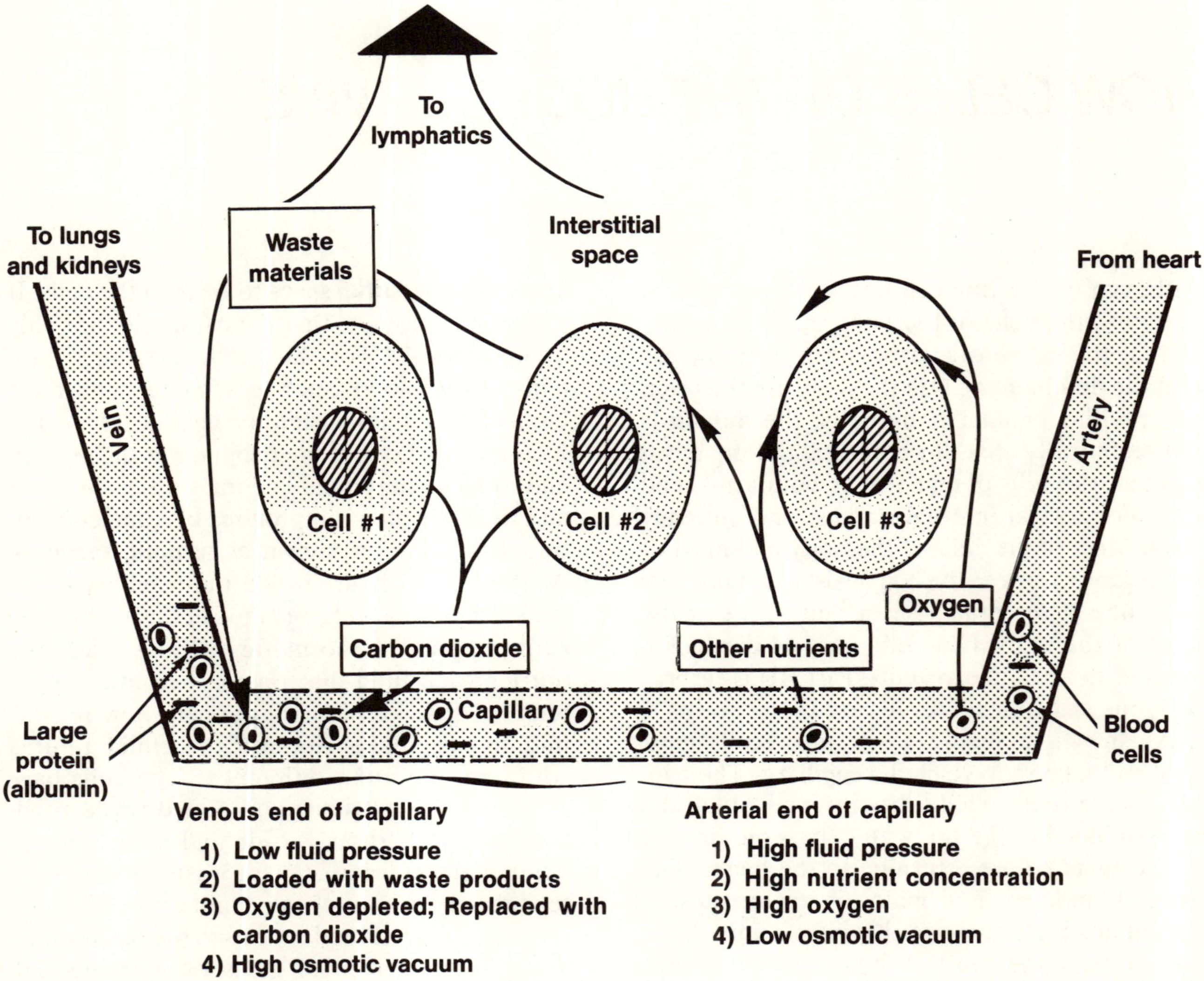

Figure 10–1. How cells in the body receive nutrients from blood vessels.

If the lymphatic drainage system becomes obstructed, if the venous capillary pressure raises too high, or if the intracapillary osmotic vacuum drops too low, an accumulation of fluid in the interstitial space will occur. This condition, known as **edema**, is discussed again in Part IV of this text.

Suggested Reading

Karp, G. *Cell Biology*. New York: McGraw-Hill, 1979.

Wolfe, S. L. *Biology of the Cell*. Belmont, CA: Wadsworth, 1981.

REVIEW QUESTIONS for How Cells of the Body Survive

1. Across which anatomical structure does nutrient exchange to the cells of the tissues take place?

Nutrient exchange takes place across the capillaries. [p. 63]

2. Name four characteristics of the blood in the arterial end of the capillary.

1) High fluid pressure
2) High in nutrients
3) High in oxygen
4) Low osmotic vacuum

[p. 63]

3. Name four characteristics of the blood in the venous end of the capillary.

1) Low fluid pressure
2) Low in nutrients, high in waste products
3) Low in oxygen, high in carbon dioxide
4) High osmotic vacuum

[p. 63]

4. Why do nutrients in the capillary circulate out to the cells in the interstitial space? Why do interstitial space waste products drain into the capillaries?

Nutrients circulate to cells in the interstitial space because high fluid pressure and low osmotic vacuum at the arterial end of the capillary forces the nutrients into the interstitial space; waste products drain into the capillaries because low fluid pressure and high osmotic vacuum at the venous end causes the waste products to return to the capillary. [p. 63]

5. How do the breakdown products from dead cells escape the interstitial space?

Dead or degraded cells are drained via the lymphatic system. [p. 63]

6. What is edema?

Edema is the accumulation of fluid in the interstitial space. [p. 64]

7. What are the three most common causes of edema?

1) Fluid pressure too high at the venous end of the capillaries.
2) Osmotic vacuum too low in the venous end of the capillaries.
3) Lymphatic system drainage obstruction.

[p. 64]

CHAPTER 11

GENETICS: INHERITANCE AND EXPRESSION OF DNA CODES

We have reviewed the biochemistry of carbohydrates, lipids, DNA, the messenger RNA that is transcribed from DNA, and the proteins for which the messenger RNA codes. We have reviewed how the ribosome translates the messenger RNA into intact proteins and how those proteins regulate the function of the cell. **Genetics** is the study of the inheritance of the specific DNA codes possessed by each cell of an organism. Genetics also explains how that set of DNA codes is expressed functionally and *which* of the total set of DNA codes are actually translated into mRNA.

DNA is divided in the nucleus into packets called **chromosomes**. Each chromosome can be thought of as one enormously long twisted ladder DNA molecule clumped into a chromosome packet. The DNA molecule in each chromosome contains the coded messages (in triplet code) for the thousands of proteins needed by the cell. As shown in Figure 11–1, the segment of a DNA molecule that codes for any single particular protein is called a **gene locus** or **gene site**. The group of nucleotide sequences that occupy a gene locus and code for one entire protein is called a **gene**. The DNA molecule in each chromosome contains thousands of genes—thousands of distinct groups of nucleotide sequences, each group coding for a different protein. Humans have *23 pairs of chromosomes* (46 twisted ladder DNA molecules) to code for all the proteins needed to create and maintain every cell in the body. Each DNA molecule has a matching DNA molecule; thus, each cell in the body (except sperm and eggs—see below) has 23 *pairs* of chromosomes, a total of 46 chromosomes. One of the 23 pairs of chromosomes codes for an individual's sex—the so-called **sex chromosomes**. The nonsex-coding genes found on the two sex chromosomes are called **sex-linked genes**. Obviously, most of the genes of each cell are found in the other 22 pairs of chromosomes; genes found on these other 44 chromosomes are called **autosomal genes**.

Although each cell in the body has all 46 chromosomes (23 matching pairs of DNA codes) in its nucleus, mature cells in the body do not have access to all of the DNA codes in their nuclei. As cells mature from their primitive embryonic form to their final adult form, they acquire specialized functions. For example, muscle cells acquire the ability to contract, nerve cells acquire the ability to conduct electricity, and B lymphocytes acquire the ability to secrete immunoglobulin. This maturation process is called **cell differentiation**. As a primitive **stem cell** differentiates into a **specialized cell**, it gains access to the nuclear DNA that codes for its specialized function; many times it will be the only cell in the body that has a particular function (and thus has access to those DNA codes). B lymphocytes are the only cells, for example, that can make immunoglobulin, and bone-forming cells are the only cells that can make bone. The rest of the DNA codes contained in the 46 chromosomes in the nucleus of every cell are covered by **DNA repressor proteins**. Because the DNA is repressed, it cannot be transcribed into mRNA and used for protein synthesis. As shown in Figure 11–2, a differentiated cell can be visualized as one that has access only to: 1) the DNA that allows it to stay alive ("house-

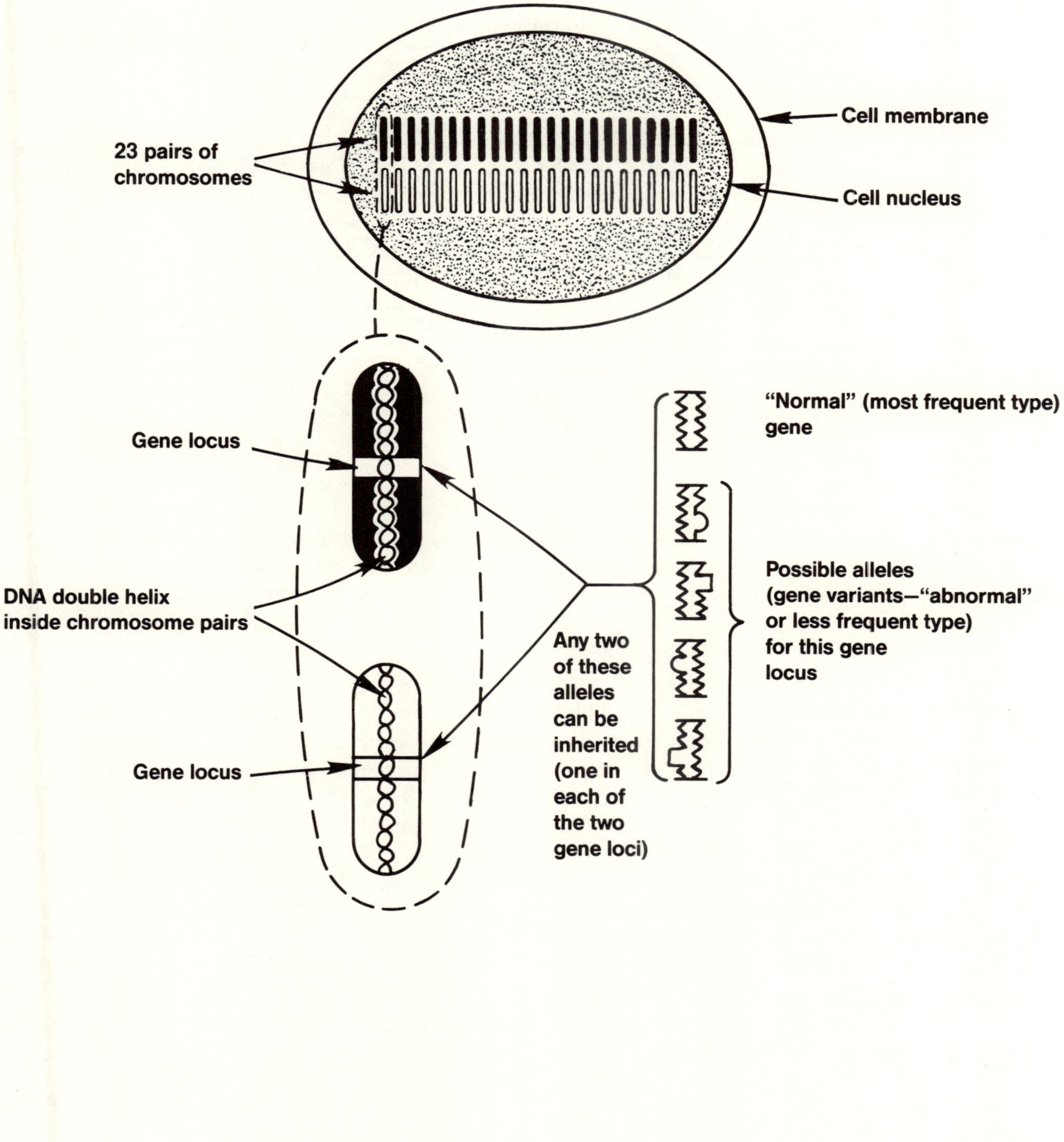

Figure 11–1. The 23 pairs of chromosomes, a gene locus on a pair of chromosomes, and the normal gene and possible alleles for that gene locus.

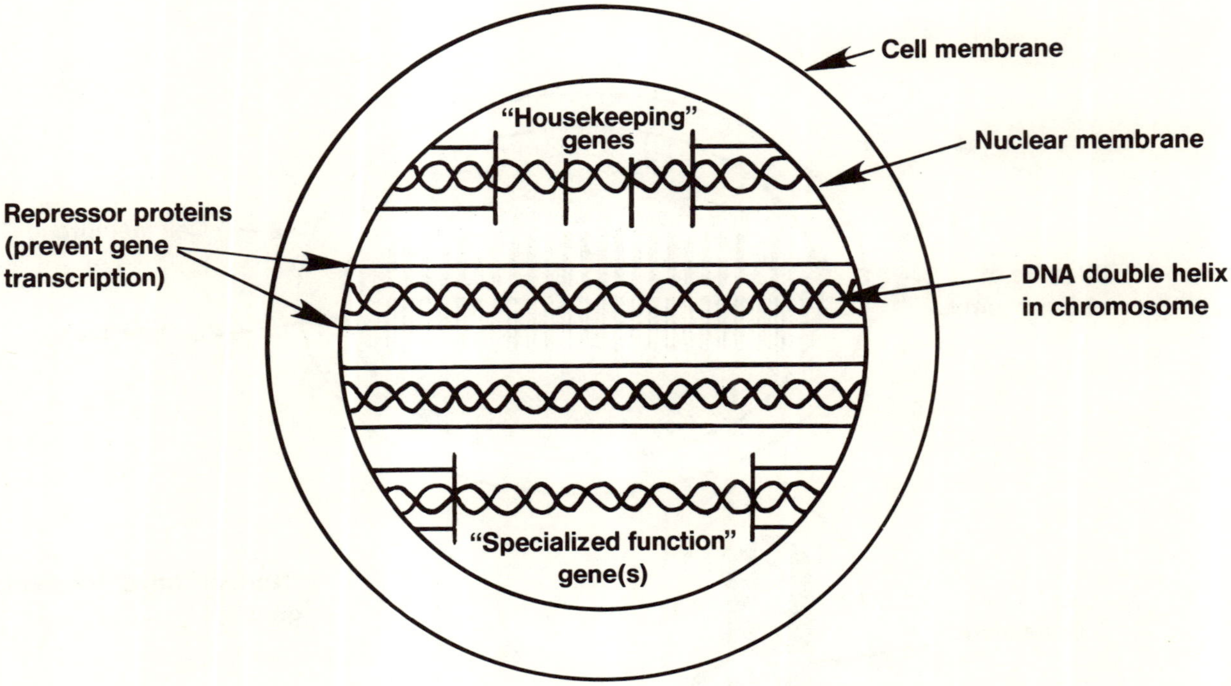

Figure 11–2. Most of the DNA ("twisted ladder" molecules) in differentiated cells is not available for gene transcription because it is covered up by represssor proteins. All cells can transcribe 1) their required "housekeeping" genes, and 2) their "specialized function" gene(s).

keeping" genes for breaking down glucose, repairing cell membranes, and so forth, which all cells need), and 2) the DNA that allows it to perform its specialized function(s). The rest of the DNA is covered with repressor proteins and is not available for use.

Each of the DNA molecules in the nucleus has a matching DNA molecule, including all housekeeping and specialized function genes. When messenger RNA (mRNA) transcripts of DNA are made, the DNA codes of both matching genes are transcribed into mRNA strands. However, mRNA can only be made from those DNA gene codes that the differentiated cell has access to (that is, not covered with repressor proteins). Often, the DNA codes at a given gene site on the two matching chromosomes are identical. Frequently however, the nucleotide sequence found in the gene locus of one chromosome is slightly different from the nucleotide sequence for the same gene found on the other matching chromosome. This event can occur when one or more DNA nucleic acid base becomes "switched" from the nucleic acid base that exists at that same site on the other matching chromosome. For example, the cytosine (C) at one point of a DNA strand might change to adenosine (A). This would mean that a triplet code message AT*C* at a certain point in the gene would change to AT*A*. This change in triplet code (from ATC to ATA) might cause a different amino acid to be inserted into the final protein assembled by the gene found on one chromosome as compared to the protein assembled from the gene found on the other matching chromosome. There are multiple mechanisms whereby such changes (**mutations**) in the DNA content of each cell can occur.

When a given gene site (the segment of DNA that contains the nucleic acid code for one entire protein) is known to have more than one DNA sequence that can occupy that gene site (thus coding for slightly different proteins) the gene site is said to have two or more **alleles**. Each *allele* is a DNA sequence that will code for a protein that is slightly different from the protein coded for by other alleles that can occupy the gene site (see Figure 11–1).

If a cell has one allele on one chromosome and a different allele on the other matching chromosome, both will be transcribed. When translated, two slightly different proteins will be made. The proteins assembled from the DNA codes of different alleles may differ by only one amino acid, as in the case of sickle cell anemia (where the sickle hemoglobin protein differs from the normal hemoglobin protein by only one amino acid). Any given gene site may be known to have hundreds of alleles (as shown from population studies), but in any one given cell there is only room for any two of those multiple alleles—one allele at the gene site of one chromosome and the same allele or a different one at the same gene site on the other matching chromosome.

One of three events can occur when a cell has two different alleles at any given gene site:

1) The cell can **coexpress** both alleles and thus express both slightly different proteins coded for by both alleles. As considered in greater detail in Chapter 22, the unique "self-code" of molecules (the **HLA system**) found on the surface of most cells of the body is derived from many coexpressive alleles found in the HLA genes of chromosome #6. These HLA molecules help define the cells of your body as being uniquely distinct from the cells of anyone else's body. Each of the two alleles that each cell inherits at each gene site is functional. Two slightly different proteins will be equally coexpressed on the cell surface.

2) Certain cell proteins (and the genes that code for them) are involved in what are called **recessive traits.** In recessive traits, a cell does not have to have two "normal" (**most frequent type**) alleles in order to function normally. One nonfunctional allele or allele that codes for a "variant" (abnormal or **less frequent type**) protein will not impair normal function. However, if a cell inherits two nonfunctional or two variant (abnormal or less frequent type) alleles, cell function will be abnormal. Abnormalities of the genetic information contained in any given cell are described at two levels: how the genetic code in that cell differs from other cells (**genotypic** variances) and how the function of the cell differs from others (**phenotypic** variances). Sickle cell anemia is one example of a recessive trait: one variant sickle hemoglobin allele produces no abnormal function (*genotypically abnormal,* but *phenotypically* [*functionally*] *normal*); two variant sickle hemoglobin alleles produce disease (*genotypically* and *phenotypically abnormal*).

3) At certain gene sites, one variant allele can **suppress** the function of the normal one; thus, if a cell inherits just one abnormal allele, it will function abnormally. This is called a **dominant trait**; in this case, a *genotypically* abnormal cell is always *phenotypically abnormal.* Huntington's chorea is an example of a dominant disease trait.

During cell division in the body's cells (**somatic cells**), called **mitosis**, all chromosomes (set ▯ and set ▮) of a cell are duplicated and passed on to the offspring cells, as shown in Figure 11–3. In contrast, during the formation of sperm or egg cells, called **meiosis**, only *one* of the two sets of chromosomes (indicated in the figure as ▯ and ▮) is passed on to each egg or sperm. As shown in Figure 11–3, there can be an **independent assortment** of each of the chromosomes of the two sets (▯ and ▮) when the two eggs or sperm are created. If the set ▯ chromosome differs at a given gene site by containing a different allele from that found in the set ▮ chromosome, one allele will go to one sperm or egg and the other allele will go to the other sperm or egg. An entire organism will be formed when the 23 chromosomes from a sperm meet the 23 chromosomes of an egg. In the process, 23 *pairs* of chromosomes are created, thus mixing the alleles found on one parent's set of 23 chromosomes with the alleles found on the other parent's set of 23 chromosomes.

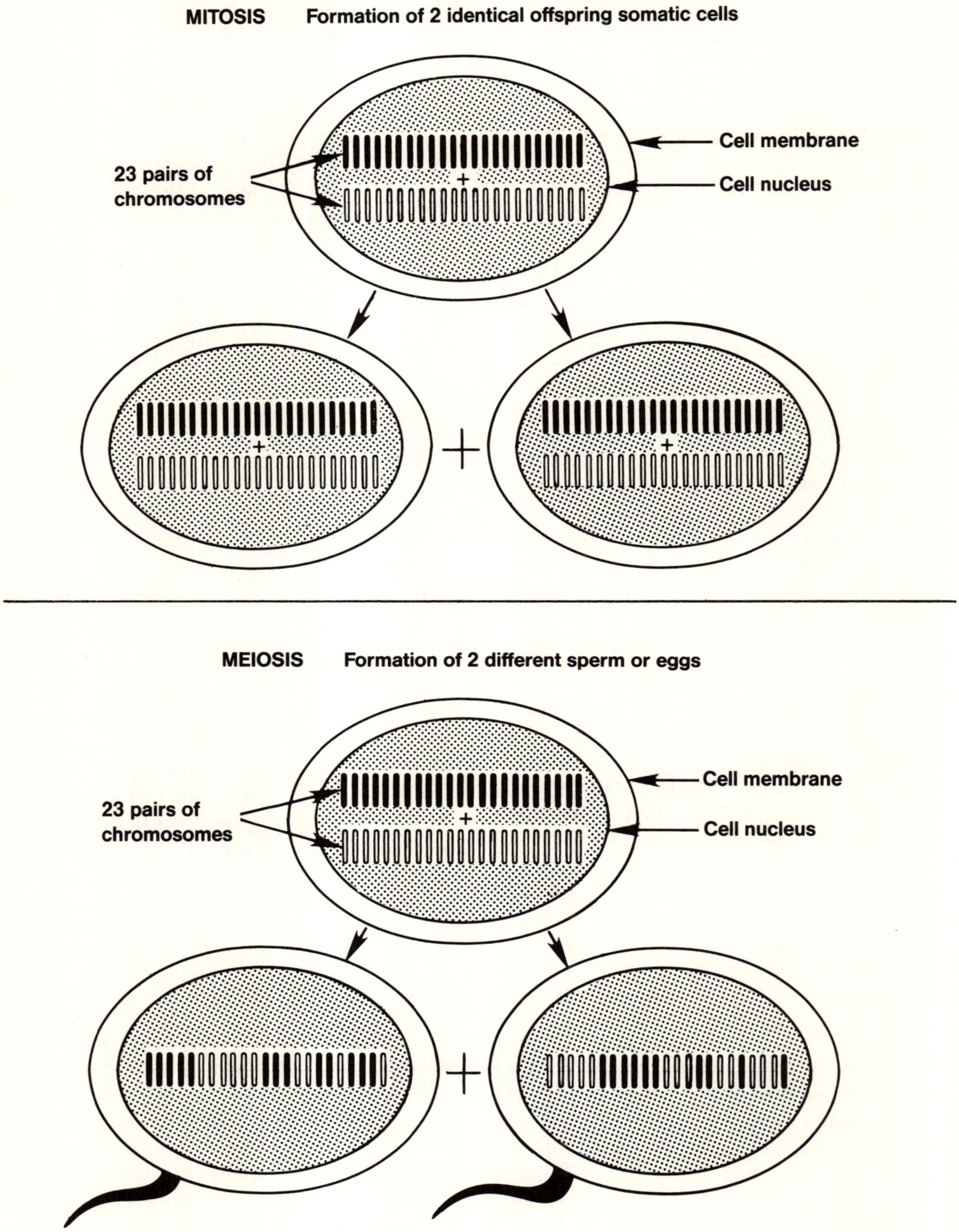

Figure 11–3. Comparison of mitosis and meiosis.

To understand the inheritance of any given trait, you must remember the following:

1) A cell has two gene sites for every protein made in the body, one on each of the two sets of chromosomes; thus, there are *two* gene sites for the trait for which the protein is responsible.
2) More than one allele may be known to exist for any given gene site.
3) No matter how many alleles are known to exist in the population for any given gene site, any single given cell can only have two. These two may be identical to one another or different.
4) If the cell has two identical normal (most frequent type) alleles at any given gene site, the cell will produce only normal proteins and have normal function (*phenotypically and genotypically normal*).
5) If the cell has two identical variant (abnormal or less frequent type) alleles at the gene site, only variant proteins will be produced and the cell will have abnormal function (*phenotypically and genotypically abnormal*).
6) If the cell has one normal allele at one gene site and one variant allele at the other matching gene site, the cell is *genotypically abnormal* but one of three functions can occur:
   a) The two alleles can *coexpress*. Both can produce proteins, each slightly different from the other, that function slightly differently. Examples of this occur in the HLA system (Chapter 22) and in the red blood cell groups (Chapter 28).
   b) If the normal allele protein product can compensate for the variant protein product, then normal cell function will occur (*phenotypically normal*); this is a *recessive trait*. It takes a double dose of the variant allele to get abnormal function in recessive traits.
   c) If the variant allele suppresses the function of the normal allele, then the cell will be *phenotypically (functionally) abnormal*. This is a *dominant trait*. One variant allele produces variant function in dominant traits.
7) A parent can only pass one allele on to his or her offspring via his sperm or her egg. If the parent has one normal and one variant allele at a given gene site, there is a 50/50 chance of passing on either the normal or the variant allele to any given sperm or egg (and thus to the progeny created by that sperm or egg).

Suggested Reading

Burns, G. W. *The Science of Genetics, An Introduction to Heredity*, 5th ed. New York: Macmillan, 1983.

Thompson, J. S. *Genetics in Medicine*, 2nd ed. Philadelphia: Saunders, 1973.

REVIEW QUESTIONS for Genetics: Inheritance and Expression of DNA Codes

1. What are chromosomes?

Chromosomes are the structures found in the cell nucleus in which each twisted ladder molecule of DNA is packeted. [p. 66]

2. How many chromosomes are in the human cell?

There are 46 chromosomes (23 pairs) in each human cell. [p. 66]

3. What is a locus?

A locus is one specific segment of a DNA molecule that codes for a single specific protein. [p. 66]

4. What is a gene?

A gene is the nucleotide sequences that occupy a locus and code for one entire protein. [p. 66]

5. How many copies of a gene exist in each cell?

Every cell has two matching sets of chromosomes. Any given gene will be found twice in each cell (once on each chromosome). [p. 66]

6. What is the difference between an autosomal and a sex-linked gene?

The sex-linked genes are found on the two sex chromosomes. The other genes, found in the other 44 chromosomes, are the autosomal genes. [p. 66]

7. What is cell differentiation?

Cell differentiation is the process whereby a cell matures and gains access to that DNA necessary for it to perform its housekeeping and specialized functions. [p. 66]

8. What is the function of DNA repressor proteins?

Repressor proteins cover those nuclear DNA codes that the cell does not need in order to perform its housekeeping or specialized functions. [p. 69]

9. What is an allele?

An allele exists when more than one set of nucleic acid sequences is known to be able to occupy any given gene site. Different alleles code for slightly different versions of the same protein product of that gene site. [p. 69]

10. What are the three possible events that can occur when a cell inherits two different alleles at a given gene site?

1) A coexpressive trait—both alleles are equally expressed.
2) A recessive trait—a cell must inherit two variant alleles in order to get variant function.
3) A dominance trait—one variant allele will suppress the function of the normal allele thus creating variant function. [p. 69]

11. What is the difference between genotype and phenotype of a cell?

Genotype refers to the actual genetic make-up (DNA sequences) found in the nucleus of the cell; phenotype refers to how the cell functions. [p. 69]

12. What is the difference between mitosis and meiosis?

Mitosis is the cell division of all body cells (somatic cells) except sperm or egg cells; offspring cells inherit all 23 pairs of chromosomes from the parent. Meiosis is the cell division that creates sperm or egg cells; offspring cells inherit only half of the 23 pairs of chromosomes (23 single chromosomes). [p. 69]

13. What are seven guidelines basic to the understanding of genetics?

1) Each cell has two matching sets of gene sites.
2) More than two alleles may exist for any given gene site.
3) Any given cell can have only two alleles.
4) If two alleles inherited are normal (most frequent type), the cell is genotypically and phenotypically normal.
5) If two variant (abnormal or less frequent type) alleles are present, the cell is genotypically and phenotypically abnormal.
6) If a cell has one normal and one variant allele, it is genotypically abnormal. Phenotype will depend on whether there is a recessive, dominant, or coexpressive pattern of allelic expression.
7) A parent can only pass on one allele to the offspring in each sperm or egg. [p. 71]

PART III

THE HUMAN IMMUNE SYSTEM

The reader is now prepared to learn about the central theme of this book, namely, the way in which the human immune system functions. The immune system is a series of specific cell types that are widely dispersed throughout the body. These cell types have available a wide range of mechanisms that allow them to repel the invasion of microorganisms and foreign substances of all kinds. The principal and classically defined function of the immune system is its specific ability to remove nonself invaders from the body. This classical description contrasts somewhat with a steadily emerging, larger definition of the immune system. The immune system is now also recognized for providing immune system homeostatis (stability of function—self regulation) as well as for protecting the body from nonself invasion. The homeostasis role of the immune system (termed the **network hypothesis**) is incompletely understood and is at the forefront of current immunology research. In Part III, the language and terminology of both the classical and the network hypotheses are reviewed to explain the human immune system function.

The immune system, unlike many other systems of the body, poses conceptual and practical problems because of its diffuse nature. Cells of the immune system are spread widely throughout the body, making it difficult to reconstruct their organization and function. Current understanding of this system is still relatively new. Several basic concepts regarding the immune system function are well established, however, and are defined here in pictorial terms for the beginning immunology student.

CHAPTER 12

OVERVIEW OF THE IMMUNE SYSTEM

The ultimate physiologic role of the immune system is to support the organ systems of the body, the most important of which is the brain. The classical vision of the immune system is of a specialized system that helps the body to distinguish self from nonself, and to eliminate nonself. Obviously, self includes everything that the body views as rightly belonging within the organism. Likewise, nonself includes any type of invasion recognized by the body as foreign, such as viral or bacterial infections, as well as the invasion of so-called "altered self" (such as *cancer*). Tumor cells, for example, were originally self cells that became detrimental to the integrity of the body. The possibility that the immune system is capable of recognizing and destroying altered self is purely hypothetical (it has never been formally proven), but this role is generally accepted as a distinct and likely possibility.

The classical purpose of the immune system is to distinguish self from nonself and to clear the nonself targets from the organism. A **target cell** is any cell that the destructive forces of the immune system are directed against. There are two components of the system: The first component deals with *recognition*. The body must be able to recognize something as nonself in order subsequently to destroy the invader. The second component deals with the actual *destruction and clearance* of the invader from the body. It is important to keep these two roles in mind. The immune system is relatively specific in its ability to recognize and clear nonself targets. The degree to which a nonself target is recognized by the immune system correlates with previous exposure of the body to that invader. For example, the immune system of a person who has been exposed to tuberculosis has been primed for that specific invader. Following reexposure to tuberculosis, an exposed person's immune response will immediately recognize and attempt to destroy the tuberculosis organism, but it will only be reactive for that particular organism (or any invader with a similar molecular make-up) and not for other nonself invaders. The immune system must be primed to respond to each particular invader that it is exposed to. It must develop immune system cells that will recognize and react to subsequent reexposure to each invader.

There are two main subsystems of the immune system that work together to recognize and remove nonself invaders. These two subsystems, as shown in Table 12–1, consist of **humoral immunity** and **cell-mediated immunity**. The humoral subsystem is basically comprised of soluble, chemical (nonliving) substances that circulate in the blood. The humoral immunity subsystem is comprised of two types of serum proteins (found in the **cell-free** liquid portion of blood). 1) **Immunoglobulins** or **Ig**, also called **antibody** molecules, provide the host with the ability to interact with *specific* nonself invaders due to the binding capacities of each antibody. Immunoglobulins (antibodies) of one type will only bind with one class of nonself molecules. These immunoglobulins are made by special white blood cells called **B lymphocytes** (to be discussed in Chapter 18). 2) **Complement components**, abbreviated as **C**, are another class of proteins in the blood used to **lyse** ("poke holes" in) nonself invaders. *The action of complement is nonspecific*. Complement must be directed to the target cell that is to be lysed. Mechanisms for this function are discussed in Chapter 19.

The *cell-mediated immunity* subsystem also has specific and nonspecific components, as shown in Table 12–1. 1) Special white cells known as **T lymphocytes** (to be discussed in Chapter

Table 12–1. The Humoral and Cell-Mediated Subsystems of Immunity.

	Humoral Immunity (consists of noncellular proteins)	***Call-Mediated Immunity (consists of living cells)***
Nonspecific in action: will attack different targets—but must be directed to do so	**Complement (C)**	**Mononuclear phagocytes PMN and NK lymphocytes**
Specific in action: will attack only one nonself target	**Immunoglobulin (Ig)**	**T lymphocytes**

17) are capable of physically confronting nonself molecules (**antigens**) and arranging for their elimination from the body. *T lymphocytes are specific*. There are many types of T lymphocytes; each type of T lymphocyte will recognize only one type of nonself invader and will not respond to other nonself invaders. 2) Other classes of white blood cells—**mononuclear phagocytes, polymorphonuclear granulocytes (PMN), and natural killer (NK) cells**—are responsible for "eating" and otherwise killing a range of nonself invaders. Thus, *mononuclear phagocytes, PMN, and NK cells are nonspecific*; they can eliminate a variety of nonself targets. This function can be amplified by signals provided by other leukocytes.

The cells that comprise the human immune system are spread throughout the body but are concentrated mainly in the body's **lymphoid system** (see Figure 12–1). This system includes the **lymphatic vessels** and **fluid**, **lymph nodes**, **spleen**, **thymus gland**, and parts of the **liver**, **lungs**, and **bone marrow**. The blood vessels of the body are a major highway used by the immune system cells to travel from one part of the immune system to any other part. The primary purpose of the lymphatic vessels is to act as a filter in clearing proteins and cells that get trapped in the interstitial spaces of the body (as reviewed in Chapter 10), and to mount an immune response to any nonself invaders found.

Most of the cells of the immune system are capable of circulating in the peripheral blood (in the arteries, capillaries, and veins) along with the other known blood cells. The cells that can be found in peripheral blood include **red blood cells** (**RBC**—they carry oxygen to tissues), **platelets** (cellular fragments responsible for blood clotting), and the **white blood cells** (**WBC**—discussed below); see also Figure 12–2. All of the cells in the peripheral blood derive or *differentiate* from a common *stem cell* found in the bone marrow. The different types of WBC constitute the immune system. As seen in Figure 12–2, WBC's can be divided into two groups: 1) **polymorphonuclear granulocytes** (**PMN**) and 2) **mononuclear leukocytes** (**MNL**). These two groups can be further subdivided into the individual cells that comprise each group. The PMN all contain **multilobed** (many lobed) **nuclei** and **cytoplasmic granules** (free-floating miniature organelles, usually containing enzymes). The three types of PMN are 1) **neutrophils**, whose granules are a pinkish color when stained, 2) **basophils**, whose granules stain dark blue, and 3) **eosinophils**, whose granules stain dark red. The PMN help defend the body nonspecifically against bacterial invasion, and thus are best conceived as part of the nonspecific, cell-mediated immune system. The MNL group is composed of two major cells, the **mononuclear phagocytes** and the **lymphocytes**. The mononuclear phagocyte is a large cell with a characteristic horseshoe-shaped nucleus. This cell is responsible for part of the nonspecific cell-mediated component of

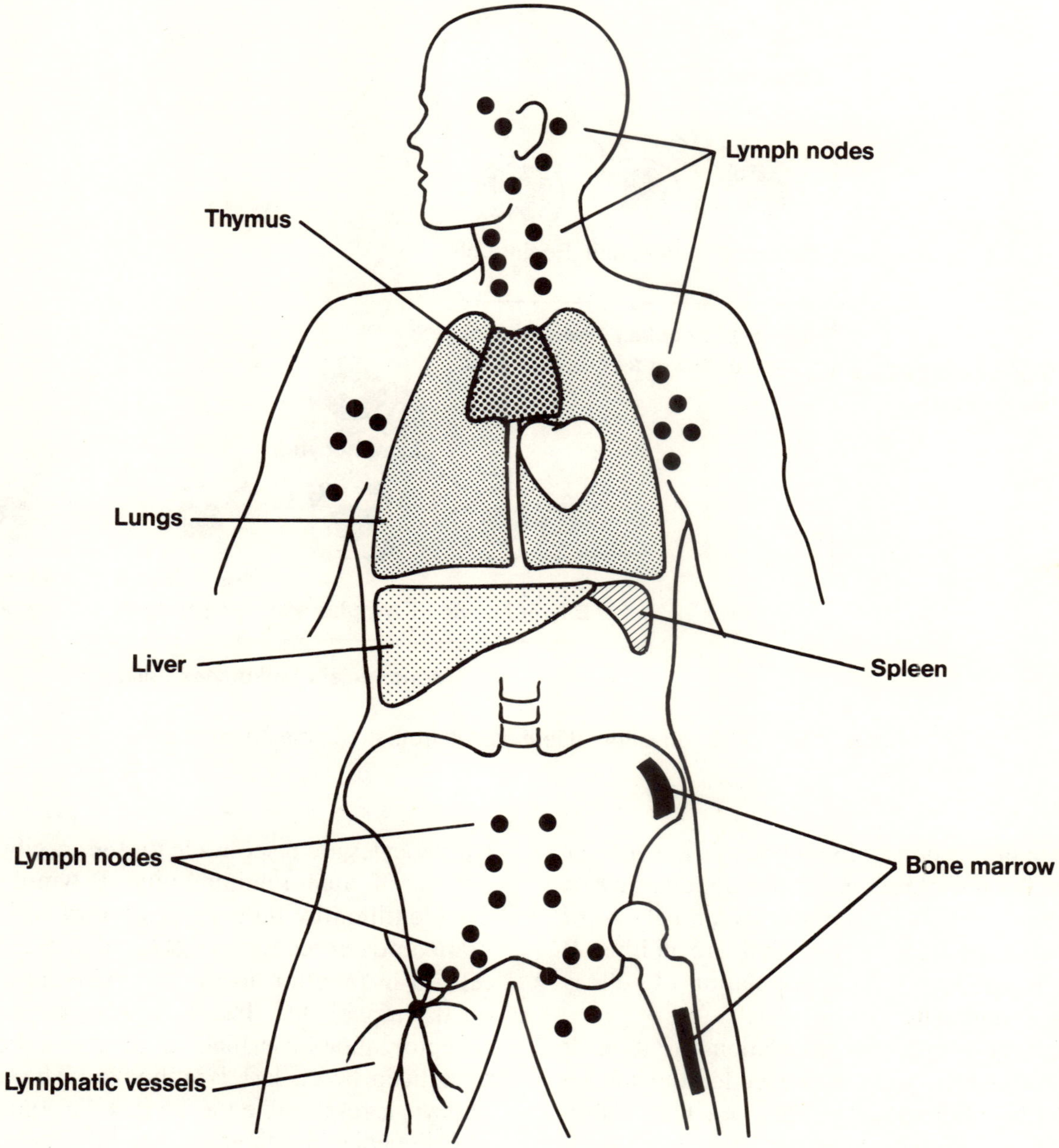

Figure 12–1. The lymphoid system.

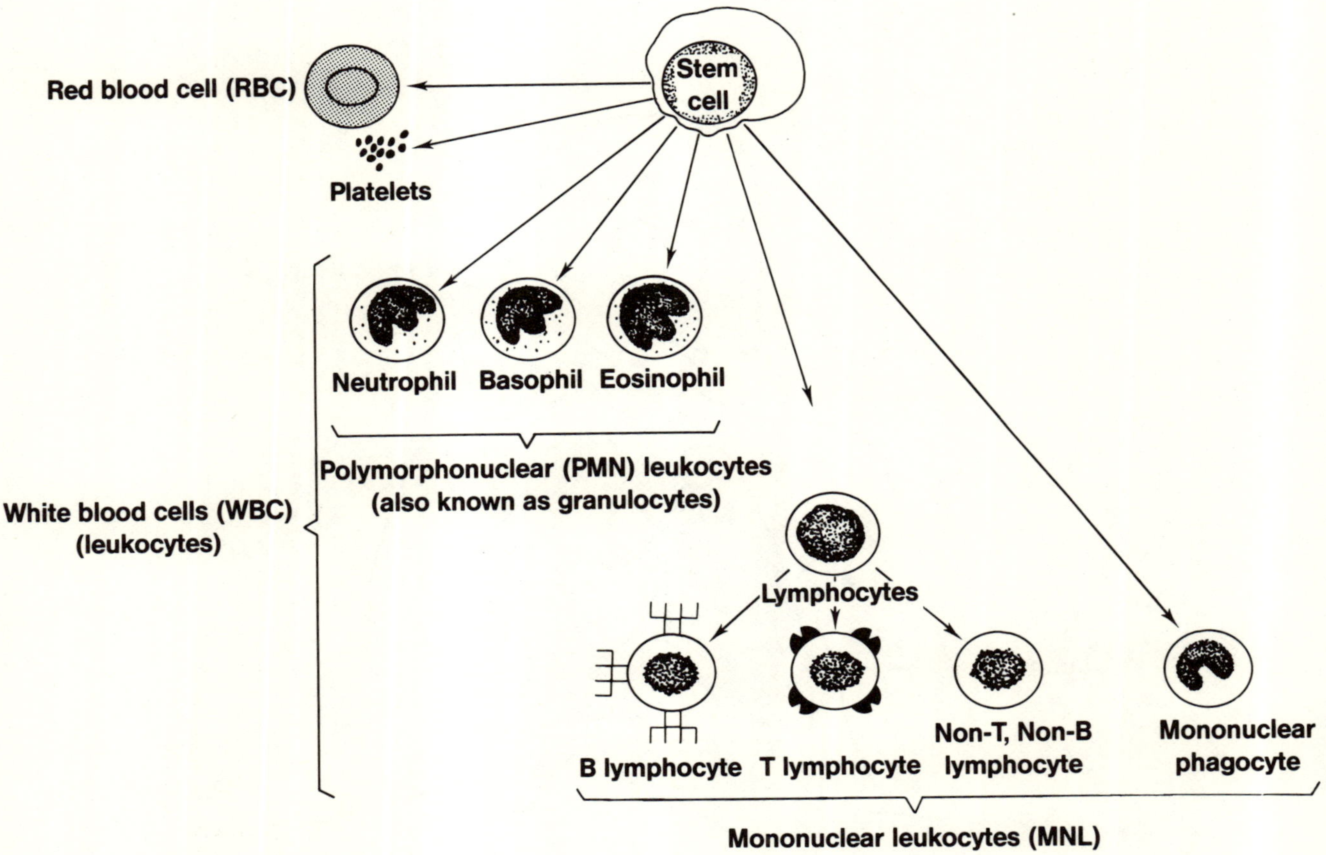

Figure 12–2. Differentiation of leukocytes from the common stem cell.

the immune response. Lymphocytes are further subdivided into three major cell populations: 1) *B lymphocytes*, 2) *T lymphocytes*, and 3) *a third population* of lymphocytes that are neither B nor T lymphocytes. This population of cells is known as **null cells**.

The three lymphocyte populations are difficult to distinguish in appearance under the microscope (morphologically). They are best distinguished functionally by what they do. The B lymphocyte is responsible for the production of immunoglobulin (Ig) proteins that bind to specific stimulating molecules called antigens (discussed in Chapter 14). The B lymphocyte is physically identified by the synthesis and expression of surface immunoglobulin (sIg;) on its cell membrane. This protein structure will recognize a specific type of nonself molecule (antigen) and will bind to it (act as a receptor). B lymphocytes are responsible for the specific component of humoral immunity. T lymphocytes are identified by their expression of cell membrane antigen-receptors ( ) that are closely related in function to the sIg molecules found on B lymphocytes. The T lymphocyte antigen-receptor allows for binding of a specific type of antigen by each T lymphocyte. The T lymphocyte is responsible for the specific component of cell-mediated immunity. The third population of lymphocytes has neither surface immunoglobulin (like B lymphocytes) nor antigen-receptors (like T lymphocytes). They are a mixed population of lymphocytes including pre-B and pre-T lymphocytes (cells that will eventually mature into B or T lymphocytes), and another cell called the natural killer (NK) lymphocyte. All of these cells and their interrelated functions are reviewed in the subsequent chapters.

The common stem cell for the lymphocytes (shown in Figures 12–2 and 12–3) is found in a particular area of the bone marrow and functions as a precursor for pre-B and pre-T lymphocytes. Lymphoid cells derived from the stem cell must migrate to one of two areas before they can mature into a functional B or T lymphocytes. B and T lymphocyte differentiation is shown in Figure 12–3. The B lymphoid cells are derived from the stem cell in the bone marrow

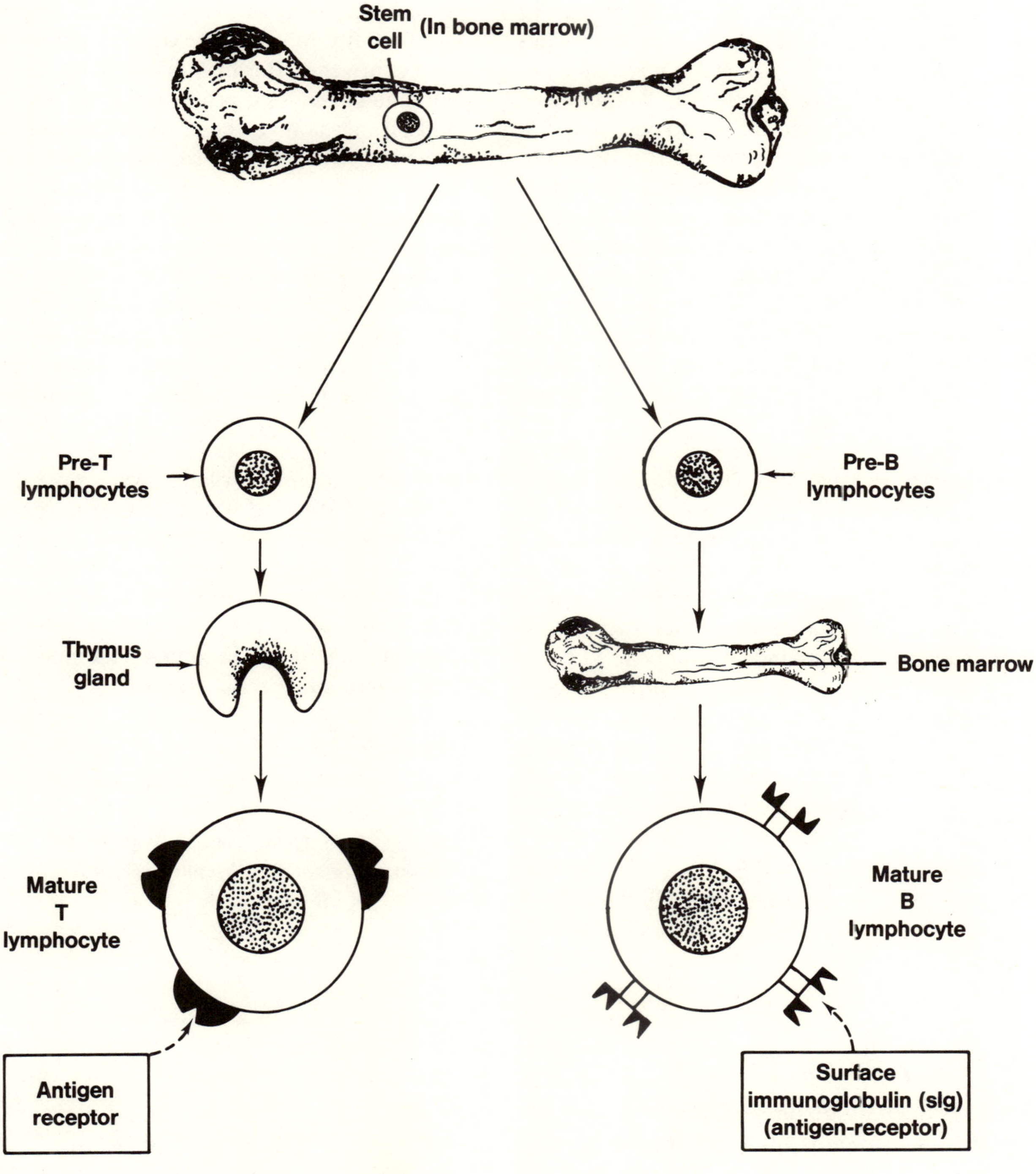

Figure 12–3. Differentiation of B and T lymphocytes.

and migrate to a different part of bone marrow where they become functional B lymphocytes. Following antigenic stimulation, the B lymphocytes are capable of being activated into **plasma cells** that will secrete immunoglobulin against the antigen. *B* lymphocytes can be thought of as referring to the fact that these cells mature in the *b*one marrow. Children who lack the particular bone marrow environment necessary for the differentiation of pre-B to B lymphocytes will not have functional B lymphocytes and will suffer from the consequence of low Ig production.

The T lymphocytes begin differentiation when their precursors migrate from the bone marrow to the thymus gland in the chest, the necessary environment for differentiation of the pre-T lymphocyte into a functional T lymphocyte. *T*-lymphocyte stands for *t*hymus-derived cell. Children born without a thymus gland do not have functional T lymphocytes and lack functional cell-mediated immunity.

It appears that the nonspecific components of immunity evolved before the specific components. That is to say, primitive animals (such as certain animals lacking backbones) have mononuclear phagocytes as their principal protection against nonself invasion. The specific components of cell-mediated immunity evolved in higher animal forms, and they appear to function as a mechanism for *amplifying and intensifying* the ability of the host to protect itself from nonself invasion. Thus, in primitive animals the principal immune response is one known as the *inflammatory response*. The primitive inflammatory response consists of migration of mononuclear phagocytes, PMN, and NK lymphocytes—the nonspecific components of cell-mediated immunity—to the site of nonself invasion. In addition to the primitive inflammatory response in higher animal forms (such as mammals), the specific B and T lymphocytes, which are capable of recognizing the particular nonself invader, are called into action and thus amplify the ability of the nonspecific components of immunity to eliminate the nonself invaders. In recent years, this classical description of the immune system as a protector of the body from nonself invasion has been somewhat expanded. Recently, the new *network hypothesis* of immune system functioning has shown that the immune system is also capable of self-regulation (homeostasis). It is thought that an additional function of the immune system is its ability to also react against self molecules when necessary to provide a smooth internal balance of immune system function. One mechanism for dampening an immune response against a nonself invader (at the appropriate time) may be to mount an additional anti-immune response *against* the first immune response, evolving into a complicated network of immune and anti-immune reactions. This *network regulation* of immune system function has been best studied with regard to the regulation of immunoglobulin secretion. We will doubtlessly learn more about the network hypothesis regarding the human immune system function in the years to come.

Suggested Reading

Eisen, H. N. *Immunology*. Hagerstown, MD: Harper & Row, 1980.

Hood, L. E., I. L. Weissman, W. B. Wood, and J. H. Wilson. *Immunology*. Menlo Park, CA: Benjamin/Cummings, 1984.

REVIEW QUESTIONS for Overview of the Immune System

1. What is the classical description of the role of the immune system?

The classical description of the role of the immune system is that it aids the body in distinguishing self from nonself (antigen) and eliminating nonself. [p. 75]

2. What are the two classical functions of the immune response?	1) Recognition of nonself 2) Elimination of nonself [p. 75]
3. What are the two main subsystems of the immune system?	1) Humoral immunity 2) Cell-mediated immunity [p. 75]
4. What are the two components of humoral immunity?	1) Complement (C) is the nonspecific component. 2) Antibodies (immunoglobulin, Ig) are the specific component. [p. 75]
5. What are the two components of cell-mediated immunity?	1) Mononuclear phagocytes, polymorphonuclear granulocytes (PMN), and natural killer (NK) lymphocytes make up the nonspecific component. 2) T lymphocytes make up the specific component. [p. 75]
6. Name the components of the lymphoid system.	Lymphatic vessels and fluid, lymph nodes, spleen, thymus gland, liver, and bone marrow. [p. 76]
7. What types of cells are found in the bloodstream?	Red blood cells (RBC), platelets, and white blood cells (WBC). [p. 76]
8. What are the two groups of white blood cells (WBC)?	Polymorphonuclear granulocytes (PMN) and mononuclear leukocytes (MNL) are the two groups of WBCs. [p. 76]
9. What are the types of polymorphonuclear (PMN) granulocytes?	Neutrophils, basophils, and eosinophils are the types of PMN granulocytes. [p. 76]
10. What are the types of mononuclear leukocytes (MNL)?	Mononuclear phagocytes and lymphocytes are MNLs. [p. 76]
11. What are the types of lymphocytes?	T lymphocytes, B lymphocytes, and third population (non-T, non-B) lymphocytes [p. 78]
12. Name the two major characteristics of T lymphocytes.	T lymphocytes have membrane antigen-receptors and are responsible for the specific component of cell-mediated immunity. [p. 78]

13. What are the two major characteristics of B lymphocytes?

B lymphocytes are responsible for immunoglobulin (Ig) production via their plasma cells and they have surface immunoglobulin (sIg) on their cell membrane. [p. 78]

14. What are the characteristics of the third population lymphocytes?

Third population lymphocytes do not have antigen-receptors or sIg. [p. 78]

15. What types of cells exist in the third population?

The natural killer (NK) lymphocytes, pre-T lymphocytes, and pre-B lymphocytes exist in the third population. [p. 78]

16. What is the definition of a B lymphocyte?

B lymphocyte is defined as a type of lymphocyte that bears sIg and is responsible for the production of Ig. They are responsible for the antigen-specific component of humoral immunity. [p. 80]

17. How was the B cell named B lymphocyte?

The B lymphocyte is derived from precursor cells that must differentiate in the bone marrow before they mature into functional B lymphocytes. [p. 80]

18. If a child is born without the bone marrow environment necessary for maturation of B lymphocytes, what will be the nature of the child's illness?

The child will lack the ability to make Ig and will suffer from the consequences of lack of specific humoral immunity. [p. 80]

19. What is the definition of a T lymphocyte?

T lymphocytes are lymphocytes that bear antigen receptors and are responsible for the antigen-specific component of cell-mediated immunity. [p. 80]

20. Why is the T lymphocyte named T lymphocyte?

The T lymphocyte is derived from precursor cells that must differentiate in the thymus gland before maturing into functional T lymphocytes. [p. 80]

21. If a child is born without a thymus gland (necessary for the maturation of T lymphocytes), what will be the nature of the child's illness?

The child will lack functional T lymphocytes and will suffer from the inability to make effective cell-mediated immune responses. [p. 80]

22. What additional immune system function is addressed in the network hypothesis?

The immune system is also capable of self-regulation (homeostasis) by reacting against certain primary immune responses. [p. 80]

CHAPTER 13

THE CLONAL NATURE OF THE IMMUNE RESPONSE

Immune responses against molecules that are perceived to be nonself (*antigens*) can be very specific. For example, a B lymphocyte will cause the production of only one kind of immunoglobulin (Ig) that will bind to and neutralize only one type of antigen. Similarly, a T lymphocyte will specifically direct the elimination of one type of nonself antigen. This specificity of the immune response is quite amazing in light of the fact that there are potentially thousands of distinct nonself antigens available. B-lymphocyte and T-lymphocyte responses can be specific for each specific class of antigens for the following reason. Just as there are thousands of types of different antigens, each person has thousands of different groups of B and T lymphocytes called **clones**—each lymphocyte clone is able to recognize only one type of antigen, that is, one type of nonself molecule.

A group of B lymphocytes that can recognize only one or more closely related antigens is known as a **B-lymphocyte clone**. A particular clone of B lymphocytes can make only one type of immunoglobulin (Ig) molecule that neutralizes only one type of antigen (or any closely related antigen). Each B-lymphocyte clone is activated to produce Ig (humoral immunity) when an antigen-specific receptor (sIg) on the surface of the B lymphocyte is stimulated by the antigen. This antigen will only stimulate those B-lymphocyte clones that have a sIg membrane molecule that can recognize and bind to the antigen. The same situation exists with **T-lymphocyte clones**. Each T-lymphocyte clone has an antigen receptor for a specific type of antigen (or any closely related antigen). When a specific antigen stimulates the appropriate T-lymphocyte clone, that clone becomes activated to neutralize the antigen, and any closely related antigens, via cell-mediated immunity.

The fact that each individual must have thousands of clones of B and T lymphocytes in order to be able to respond to the thousands of different types of nonself antigens helps to explain why there is a period of about 1–3 weeks (lag time) following **primary exposure** before maximal amounts of specific immune responses are made. In the 1–3 weeks following primary exposure, the small numbers of antigen-specific B- and T-lymphocyte clones expand (proliferate) to promote the destruction of the antigen. The initial expansion of a clone simply involves multiple cell replication known as **clonal proliferation** (Figure 13–1). Each one of the offspring cells shares the antigen specificity of the parent clone cell. This process can take 1–3 weeks. In addition (as discussed in Chapters 14 and 15), primary exposure to each antigen stimulates the development of memory B- and T-lymphocyte clones for the antigen. These memory B and T lymphocytes remain "at the ready" long after the primary exposure and antigen elimination is complete. The process of clonal proliferation, following antigenic stimulation, and the development of memory B and T lymphocytes is known as **immunization**.

Immune responses following secondary exposure to an antigen occur more rapidly and are larger in magnitude. The antigen-specific B- and T-lymphocyte memory cells have memory for the antigen. Clonal proliferation occurs much faster during subsequent exposures than following the primary exposure. Specific elimination of antigen by the immune system is much more

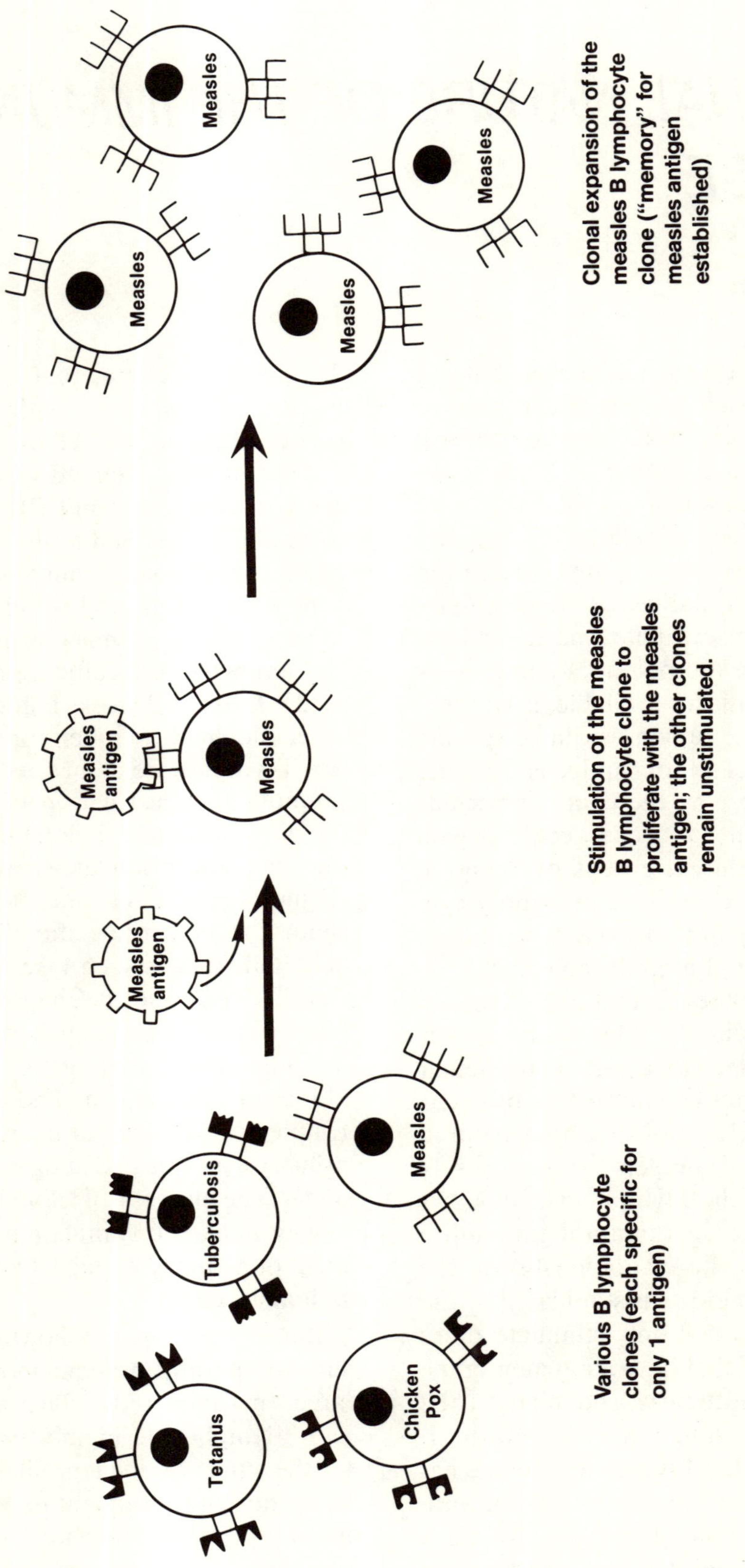

Figure 13–1. Clonal expansion of the measles B-lymphocyte clone following exposure to the measles antigen.

rapid (it can begin within 1–3 days) and is efficient in an immunized individual (following secondary exposure).

Suggested Reading

Kabat, E. A. *Structural Concepts in Immunology and Immunochemistry*. New York: Holt, Rinehart & Winston, 1976.

Stites, D. P., J. D. Stobo, H. H. Fudenberg, and J. V. Wells. *Basic and Clinical Immunology*, 4th ed. Los Altos, CA: Lange Medical Publications, 1982.

REVIEW QUESTIONS for The Clonal Nature of the Immune Response

1. What is an antigen?

An antigen is a molecule perceived as being nonself by the immune system. [p. 83]

2. To how many antigens can a clone of B or T lymphocyte respond?

One lymphocyte responds to one antigen (or certain closely related antigens). [p. 83]

3. What is a lymphocyte clone?

A lymphocyte clone is a group of B or T lymphocytes that is committed to respond to only one type of antigen. [p. 83]

4. What is immunization?

Immunization is the process of primary exposure of a lymphocyte clone to its stimulating antigen so that the clone can undergo proliferation and acquire memory for the antigen—the priming of the immune response. [p. 83]

5. How long is the lag period before a maximal specific immune response occurs after primary immunization?

There is a period of 1–3 weeks (lag time) following primary exposure before a maximal specific immune response occurs. [p. 83]

6. How long is the lag period before a specific immune response occurs following secondary immunization? Why?

Secondary immunization response occurs within a much shorter period (beginning within 1–3 days) because the immune system has been primed. The B- and T-lymphocyte clones now have memory for that antigen. [p. 83]

CHAPTER 14

THE NATURE OF IMMUNOGLOBULINS: STRUCTURE AND FUNCTION

Immunoglobulins (Ig) (antibodies) are proteins, produced by B lymphocytes, which are capable of binding to specific nonself molecules (*antigens*). Each Ig protein can be visualized three-dimensionally as a lobster, with the two claws representing the antigen-binding portion. The back part of the Ig, analogous to the tail of the lobster, does not bind antigen (see Figure 14–1).

Each Ig molecule is composed of four polypeptide chains that are linked by disulfide (–S–S–) bridges. There are two polypeptide chains called light (L) chains and two polypeptide chains known as heavy (H) chains. One obvious difference between the L chains and the H chains is the fact that the H chains are about two to two and one-half times as long as the L chains and are thus heavier. There are several other differences between the L and H chains.

As shown in Figure 14–2, the two L chains consist of roughly two halves. The portion of the L chain in the hind portion of the lobster claw, the **constant region**, is composed of two main types of amino acid sequences: lambda (λ) or kappa (κ) light chain sequences. This portion of the L chain can be only one type of amino acid sequence (the lambda [λ] sequence) or the other type (the kappa [κ] sequence). This portion of the L chain is called the *constant region* because only two main types of amino acid variations exist. In any given Ig the constant region of the two L chains will always be identical—either λ or κ, never a combination of the two. The other half of each L chain (towards the front of the lobster claw) is known as the **variable (V) region**. The amino acid sequences in the variable region of the L chains will vary from immunoglobulin to immunoglobulin because this is the area of the L chain which contributes to the binding site for antigen. There are literally thousands of different antigens, so there must be thousands of different types of amino acid sequences of the variable (V) regions in the L chains to be able to bind to this diversity of antigens.

The H chains have a variable (V) region that is approximately as long as the V regions of the L chains (110–120 amino acids). The variable (V) region of the H chains contributes the other half of the binding site for antigen. The amino acid sequences of the H chain V region will usually be different from those found on the L chain V region. The constant (C) region of the H chains is much longer than the constant region of the L chains. Note that the constant region of the L chain is approximately 110 amino acids long, whereas the constant region of the H chains is usually three to four times longer.

When the amino acid sequences of the constant regions of H chains are analyzed, five general classes of amino acid sequences can be found, as opposed to the two types (κ and λ) in the L chains. These five types of amino acid sequences of the H chains determine the class of the Ig. The five known classes of Ig are called Ig*G*, Ig*A*, Ig*M*, Ig*E*, and Ig*D*. The letters G, A, M, E, and D come from Greek words used to name the H chain type of that Ig. The H chains are denoted as 1) **gamma** (γ, IgG), 2) **alpha** (α, IgA), 3) **mu** (μ, IgM), 4) **epsilon** (ϵ, IgE), and 5) **delta** (δ, IgD). All H chains fall into one of these five general classes of amino acid sequences (although minor variants called subclasses are

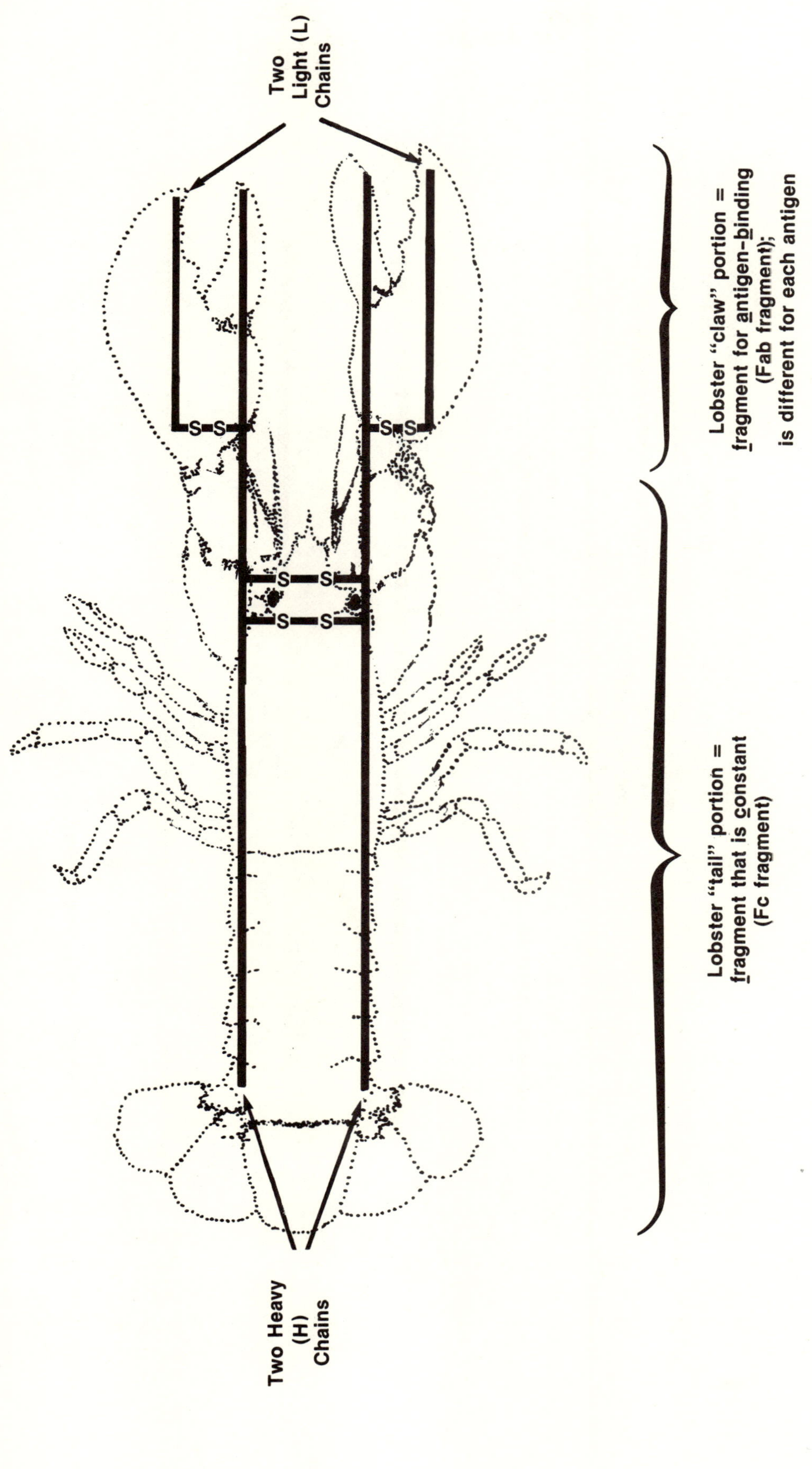

Figure 14–1. Analogy between an immunoglobulin and a lobster.

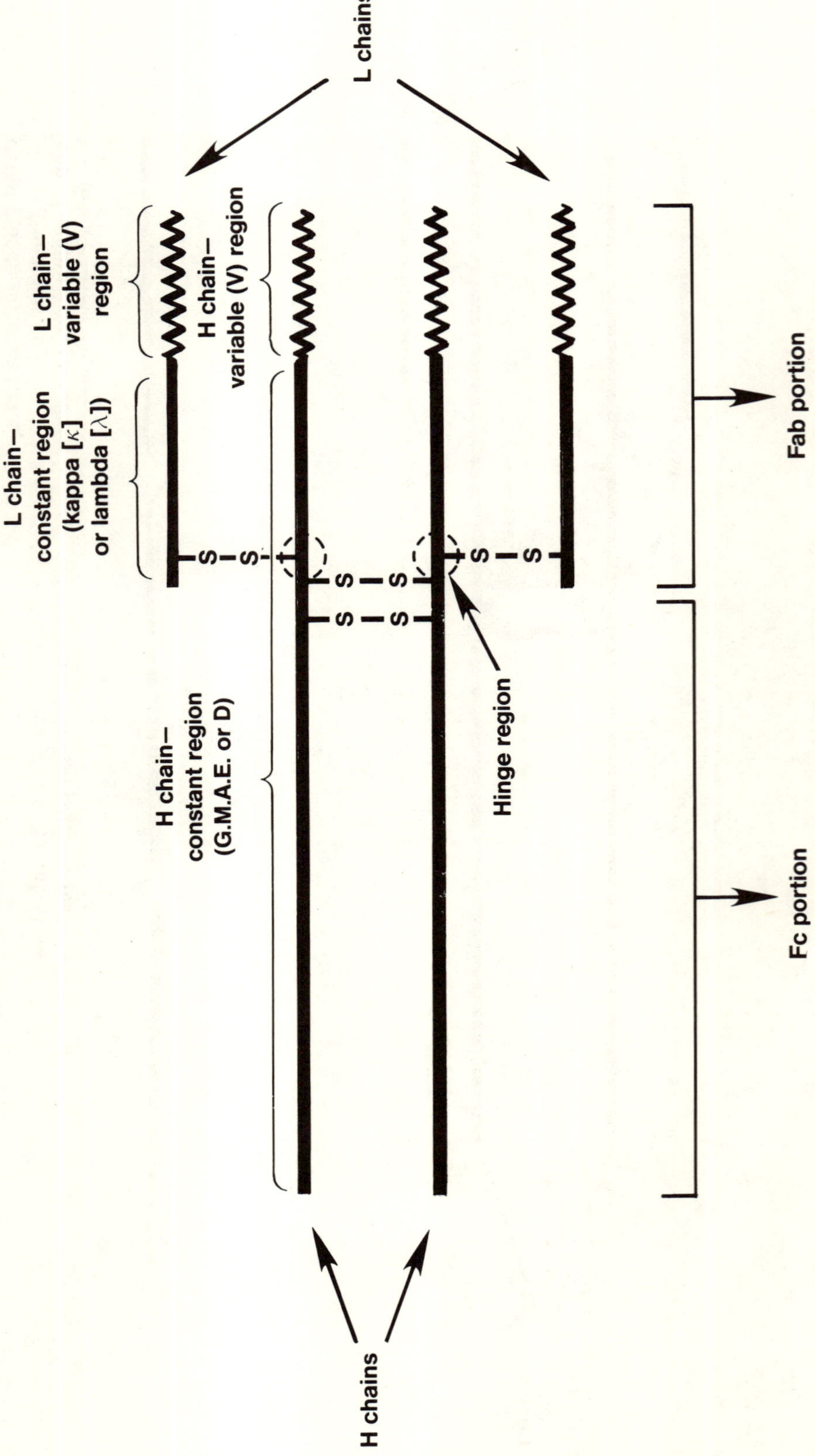

Figure 14–2. Component parts of an immunoglobulin molecule.

known to exist). Therefore, all Ig falls into one of the five known classes on the basis of their H chain amino acid sequence.

The portion of the Ig that makes up the entire lobster claw is called the **Fab region** (*f*ragment for *a*ntigen *b*inding). The rest of the Ig (lobster tail portion) is called the **Fc region** (*f*ragment that is *c*onstant [can also be concentrated into *c*rystals]). The two regions of Ig possess distinct, yet interrelated, functions. The area of the immunoglobulin molecule between the Fab portion (lobster claw) and Fc portion (lobster tail) is called the **hinge region** (Figure 14–2). This region is flexible and allows for greater mobility of the Fab region (allows the claw to move).

The Fab fragment is the exclusive antigen-binding portion of immunoglobulin. Antigen binding occurs via the unique amino acid sequences of the two terminal V regions of the L and H chains. The differences between the V region of the H and L polypeptide chains are the R groups found on the various individual amino acids that make up each chain (Chapter 5). The major activity of these R groups relates to their size and the electrical charge that each possesses. Thus, the Fab V region can be visualized as having different sized and distinctly charged particles (R groups) sticking out from the L and H chains. To return to the lobster analogy, the teeth of the lobster claw portion of the Fab fragment are simply the R groups of the various amino acids that make up the V regions of the L and H chains. The antigen will bear certain polar groups that have electrical charges and distinct sizes as well (especially protein antigens, but other biomolecules too). The electrical charges on the antigen will be attracted to the electrical charges of the Fab regions if the charges are opposite and the sizes of the interacting R groups are compatible. As shown in Figure 14–3, the antigen will be held in the Fab region primarily by electrical attraction. No covalent bonding is involved. Other forces may contribute to protein antigen binding by the Fab region, but electrical attraction between compatible sized R groups is the principal force.

Ig (antibody) structure is not, in fact, straight (the primary sequence structure) as is shown in the schematic drawing of Figure 14–2. The structure is actually globular (the tertiary structure) such that the number of amino acids that actually comprise the antigen-binding area is very small. The antigen-binding site is so small that it can hold only about six amino acids of any given protein antigen molecule. A typical complex antigen (such as a bacterium) may be made up of hundreds of distinct separate antigens known as **epitopes** and, thus, hundreds of different Ig can bind to it.

When a single epitope is injected into an animal, a group of B lymphocytes (a group of B-lymphocyte *clones*) whose antibodies react with the epitope will become activated. These B-lymphocyte clones will react, proliferate, and transform into Ig-secreting cells called *plasma cells*. In addition, the B-lymphocyte clones will develop memory cells for that antigen. The Ig made by each B-lymphocyte clone will bind to the antigen. If a complex antigen (most antigens are very big, having many distinct antigens [epitopes]) is injected into a laboratory animal, many clones of B lymphocytes will respond—a **polyclonal response**. The different clones of B lymphocytes will each secrete a different Ig, making **polyclonal antibodies** (an array of many different Ig molecules from many different clones). If large amounts of a single immunoglobulin molecule, called a **monoclonal antibody**, are desired, each distinct B-lymphocyte clone in the spleen of the laboratory animal must be separated from the other and fused with an immortal malignant (cancer-like) B lymphocyte (see Figure 14–4). Proliferation of these new hybrid cells, called **hybridomas**, takes place in special test tubes called tissue culture flasks. The result of the proliferation is a huge number of Ig-secreting hybridoma cells that are all of one clone. Thus, the monoclonal antibodies produced will be homogenous, that is, identical. Development of monoclonal antibodies represents an exciting approach to understanding how B lymphocytes work. They are currently being used in clinical trials for the treatment of

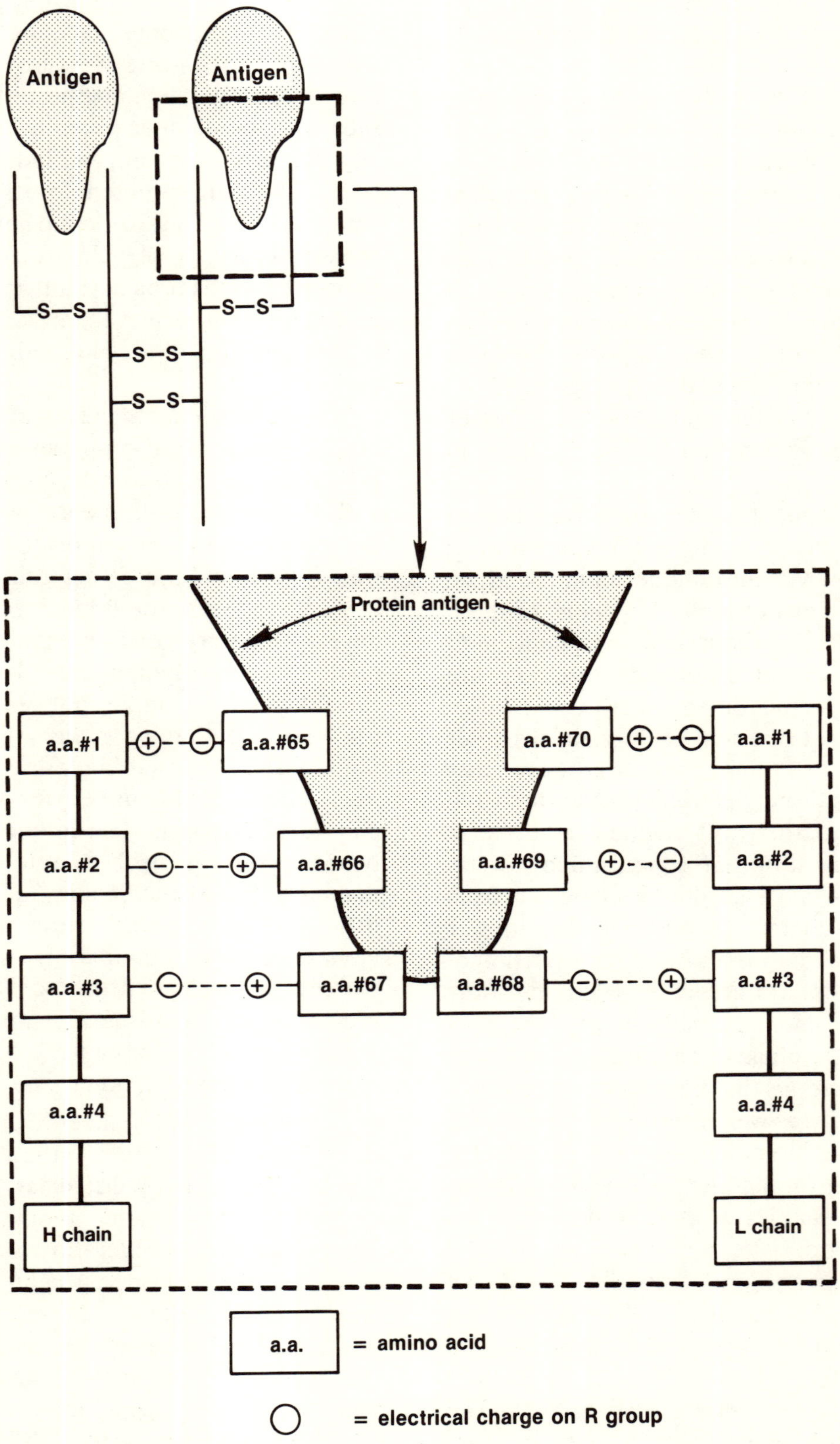

Figure 14–3. How electrical attractions between the R groups of immunoglobulin and protein antigen hold the antigen into the antigen-binding site.

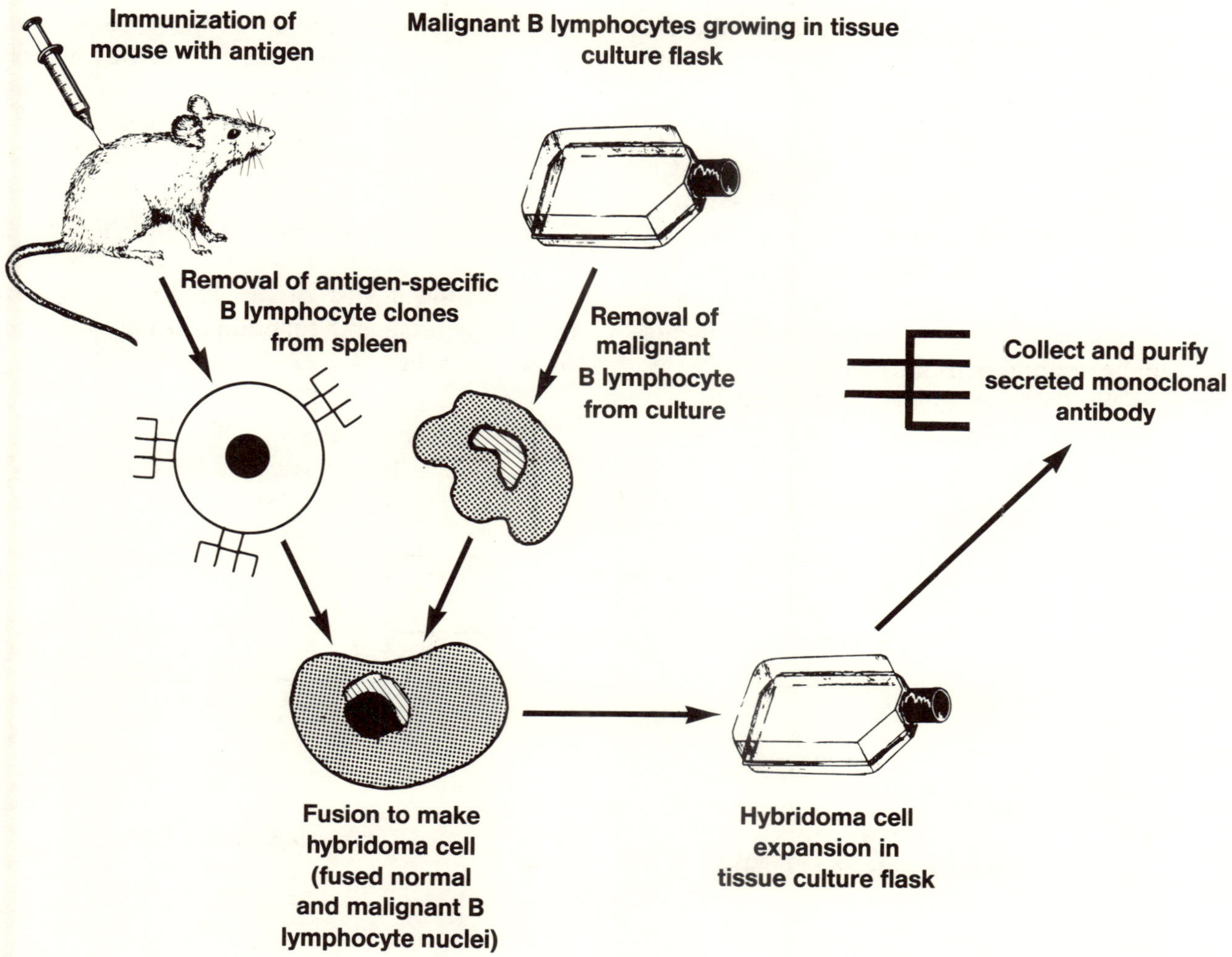

Figure 14–4. Steps involved in the formation of monoclonal antibodies.

cancer patients and as diagnostic reagents (laboratory materials) to detect human disease states (Part IV).

Once the concept of **clonality** is understood, the concept of **idiotype** will be clear. Idiotype pertains to the structure of the antigen-binding V regions of the L and H chains of Ig (teeth of the lobster claw) that is produced by any given B-lymphocyte clone. When we mention the idiotype structure we are referring to *the specific, known amino acid sequence, the primary structure, of any given Ig* antigen-binding V region. If the exact amino acid sequence of the antigen-binding site of an Ig molecule can be replicated, its idiotype has been replicated. By definition, all Ig of a given B-lymphocyte clone are of the same idiotype, that is, they are identical Ig with identical antigen-binding properties. Recall that the membrane receptor for antigen for each B-lymphocyte clone is Ig. Each B lymphocyte has Ig on its surface (sIg), which binds to a specific antigen. This binding event is a B-lymphocyte activation signal. The sIg on the surface of each B lymphocyte is the same idiotype of Ig that the B lymphocyte will secrete following activation.

The Fc portion of Ig (the lobster tail portion) determines a number of the functional properties of the Ig. Note that when Ig binds to live cell antigens (such as bacteria), it does *not* destroy the antigen; Ig binding may hinder a nonself cell but in no way kills it. There must be other mechanisms that cause the final destruction of live cell antigens. Two mechanisms that perform this function are: 1) the **complement system**—nonspecific humoral immunity components, and 2) recruitment of cells that have receptors for the Fc portion of Ig—monocytes, PMN, and NK lymphocytes—the nonspecific components of cellular immunity. Both mechanisms are described in greater detail later in this text.

Nonliving antigens (nonself molecules such as drugs and poisonous toxins) can be neutralized by reacting them with Ig that is specific for each antigen. These **antigen–antibody complexes** can then be ingested and cleared from the body by Fc receptor-bearing killer cells as described above. Several diseases can occur from breakdown of this clearance mechanism, as described later in Part IV.

The following list of the Ig classes reviews their structural and functional differences (as shown in Figure 14–5):

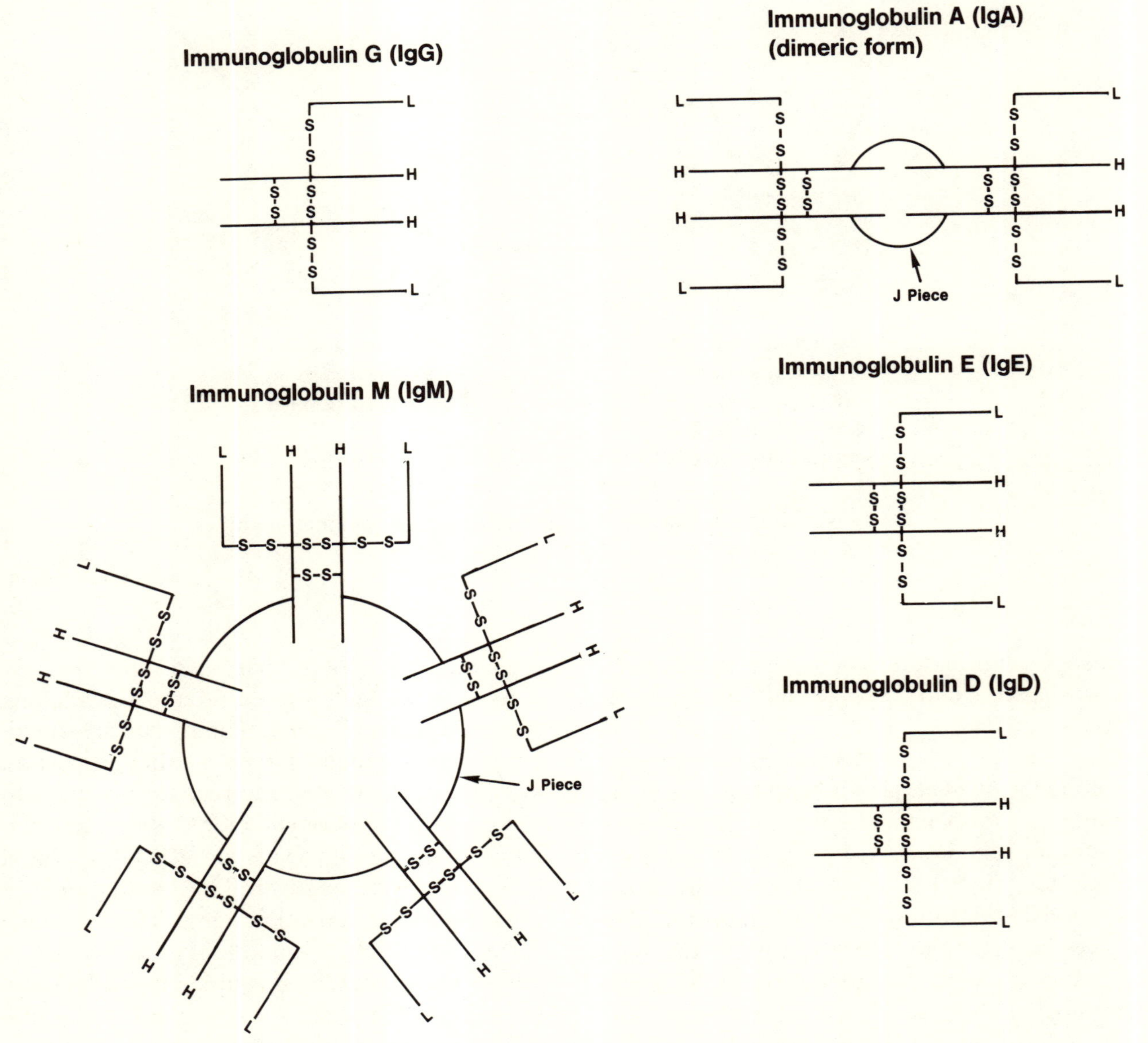

Figure 14–5. Examples of the five classes of immunoglobulins.

IgG (*monomeric*) is the classic Ig type of molecule. It has a molecular weight of approximately 150,000 (grams/mole). It is able to *activate complement (C)*. IgG is only released in significant amounts into the bloodstream after *secondary exposure to antigen*. Also, it is the only immunoglobulin that can cross the placenta (give *passive immunity* from the mother to the newborn).

IgM (*pentameric*) is able to *activate C*. It has a molecular weight of approximately 950,000. It is the first Ig class to appear in the bloodstream against any given antigen upon *primary exposure* to antigen. Its five components are held together by a *j*oining (J) piece; each IgM molecule has more antigen-binding sites than IgG.

IgA (has both *monomeric* and *dimeric* forms) is found in most secretions such as milk, tears, and intestinal secretions. Therefore, IgA is the first line of defense against invasion from bacteria and viruses trying to penetrate the mucous membranes. The monomeric form of IgA has a molecular weight of approximately 160,000. In the dimeric form (molecular weight = 405,000), the two components of IgA are held together by a joining (J) piece. IgA *does not activate C*.

IgE (*monomeric*) is produced mainly in allergic individuals and is responsible for most-allergic symptoms. It is also produced in response to parasitic infestation. Its molecular weight is approximately 200,000. IgE *does not activate C*.

IgD (*monomeric*) is mainly found on the surface of B lymphocytes (sIg). Its molecular weight is about 180,000. Little is known about the function of this Ig.

Suggested Reading

Hood, L. E., I. L. Weissman, W. B. Wood and J. H. Wilson. *Immunology*. Menlo Park, CA: Benjamin/Cummings, 1984.

Kabat, E. A. *Structural Concepts in Immunology and Immunochemistry*. New York: Holt, Rinehart & Winston, 1976.

REVIEW QUESTIONS for The Nature of Immunoglobuins

1. What are immunoglobuins (Ig)?

Ig are proteins produced by B lymphocytes. They are capable of binding to specific antigens. (Immunoglobulins are also known as antibodies.) [p. 86]

2. What are the names of the four polypeptide chains that make up an Ig?

Light (L) chains (2) and heavy (H) chains (2) make up an Ig. [p. 86]

3. How are those chains covalently held together?

Polypeptide chains are held together by disulfide bonds. [p. 86]

4. How many types of light chains are there?

There are two types of light chains: kappa and lambda light chains. [p. 86]

5. How are the light chain types determined?

The light chain types are determined by the amino acid sequence of their constant portion. [p. 86]

6. What are the two main regions of an Ig?

The two main regions of an Ig are the antigen-binding, variable regions of the L and H chains (found in the Fab region), and the constant region of the H chains (Fc portion). [p. 86]

7. What is the function of the variable region?

The variable region binds antigen. [p. 86]

8. How many Ig heavy chains classes exist?

Five types of heavy chain classes exist. [p. 86]

9. How is the heavy chain class determined?

The class is determined by the amino acid sequence it possesses. There are five known general classes of heavy chain types. [p. 86]

10. What are the five classes of Ig?

Heavy chain	Immunoglobulin class name
Gamma	IgG
Alpha	IgA
Mu	IgM
Epsilon	IgE
Delta	IgD

[p. 86]

11. Name the five classes of heavy chains.

1) Gamma (γ)
2) Alpha (α)
3) Mu (μ)
4) Epsilon (ϵ)
5) Delta (δ) [p. 86]

12. How is the immunoglobin (Ig) class determined?

The class is determined by the kind of heavy chain each Ig possesses. [p. 86]

13. What does the tail of the lobster represent?

The tail represents the Fc region. [p. 89]

14. How are the Fab and Fc regions of the Ig held together?

They are held together by a flexible hinge region. [p. 89]

15. In the comparison of one Ig molecule with a lobster, what do the claws of the lobster represent?

The claws represent the Fab region. [p. 89]

16. What is the function of the Fab region?

The function of the Fab region is to bind antigen (antigen-binding fragment). [p. 89]

17. How is an antigen held in the Fab region?

An antigen is held principally by electrical attractions and size interactions between the R groups of the variable regions of the light and heavy chains, and the electrical charges and size of molecular structures that exist on the antigen. [p. 89]

18. What is a monoclonal antibody?

A monoclonal antibody is an immunoglobulin produced by one single clone of a B lymphocyte; thus, all the monoclonal antibody (Ig) molecules will have identical structures. [p. 89]

19. What is an idiotype?

An idiotype is a specific, known primary amino acid sequence of the antigen-binding site (V region of the L and H chains) of an Ig. (If two Ig are identical in their antigen-binding region amino acid sequence, they have the same idiotype and, thus, the same antigen-binding characteristics.) [p. 91]

20. What two mechanisms are available for destruction of a live cellular antigen that is bound by an Ig molecule?

1) The complement system and 2) the presence of Fc receptor bearing killer cells that will kill the antibody-coated target. [p. 92]

21. How are small nonliving antigenic molecules cleared from the body?

Specific Ig will bind to the antigen molecule and neutralize it. Then the antigen–antibody complex can be cleared by Fc receptor-bearing killer cells. [p. 92]

22. What are the basic characteristics of IgG?

IgG is monomeric and is capable of activating complement (C). It will only be made following secondary exposure to an antigen. It is the only immunoglobulin that can cross the placenta. [p. 93]

23. What are the basic characteristics of IgM?

IgM is pentameric, and thus can bind antigen most efficiently. It is able to activate C, and is the first Ig class synthesized after primary exposure to an antigen. [p. 93]

24. What are the basic characteristics of IgA?

IgA can be either monomeric or dimeric in form. It is found in most bodily secretions, and is the first line of defense against microbes invading through the mucous membranes. [p. 93]

25. What are the basic characteristics of IgE?

IgE is monomeric, is prevalent in allergic individuals, and is responsible for most allergic symptoms. It is also produced in patients reacting to parasitic infestation. [p. 93]

26. What are the basic characteristics of IgD?

IgD is monomeric and is found on the surface B lymphocytes; little else is known about its function. [p. 93]

CHAPTER 15

THE COMPONENTS OF THE IMMUNE RESPONSE

Four components of the immune response have been introduced in previous chapters: specific and nonspecific components of humoral immunity, and specific and nonspecific components of cell-mediated immunity. These components are now described in detail in the context of the overall immune response. Before we proceed, however, it is necessary to introduce one additional component—**antigen processing**. These five components and their complicated interrelationships are depicted in Figure 15–1. Please do not be alarmed at the complexity of this very important schematic; each element of the figure is described in detail in the following order:

1) Antigen processing
2) T-lymphocyte activation (cell-mediated immunity, specific component)
3) B-lymphocyte activation (humoral immunity, specific component)
4) Complement activation (humoral immunity, nonspecific component)
5) Role of mononuclear phagocytes, polymorphonuclear leukocytes (PMN), and natural killer (NK) cells (cell-mediated immunity, nonspecific component)

Each of the next five chapters is devoted to one of the above components of the overall immune system schematic. The relevant section of the overall schematic discussed in each chapter is presented immediately below the chapter title. Each aspect of this critical figure is described in detail. At the end of this review all of the component parts of the figure are reassembled in order that you can absorb the entire figure.

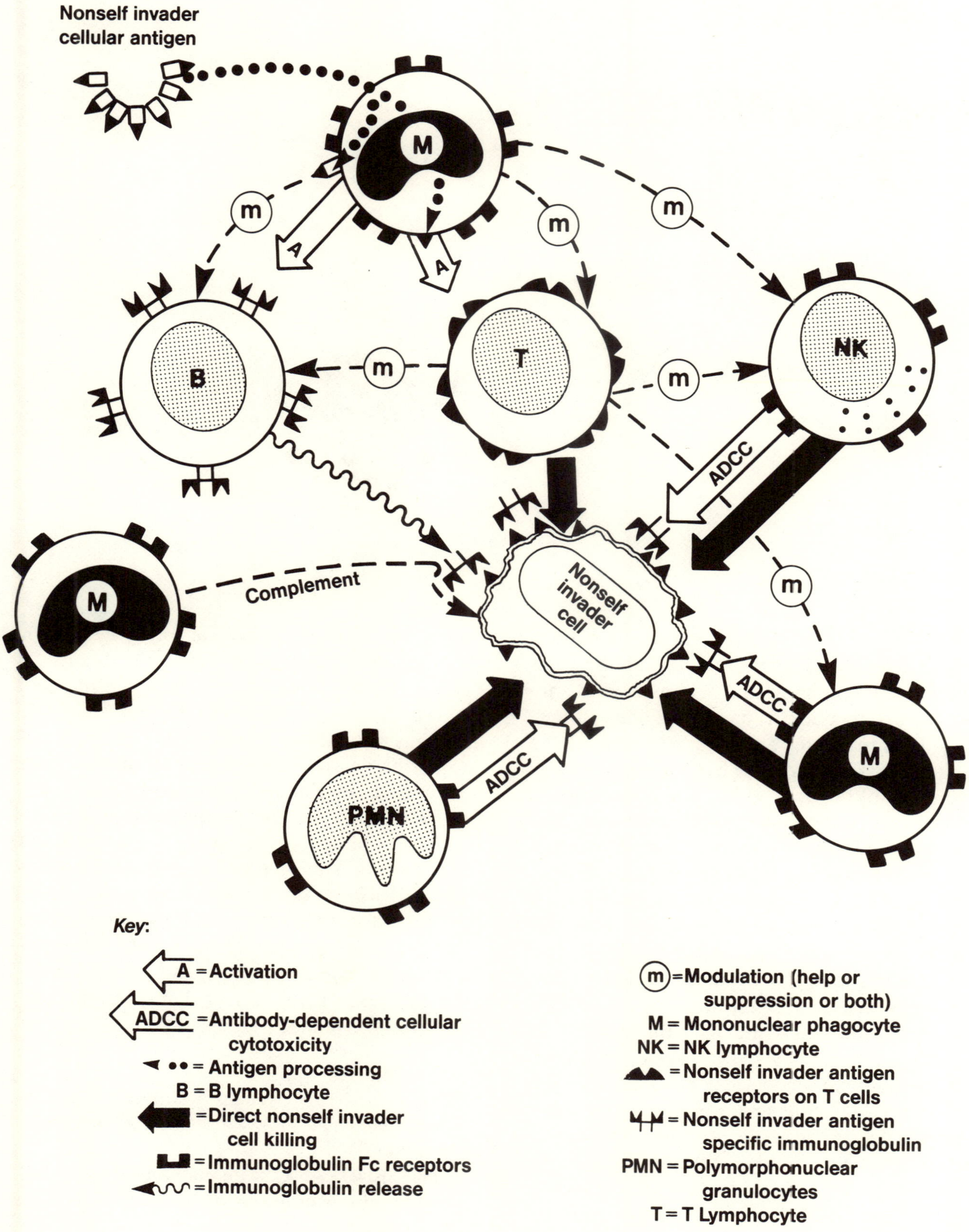

Figure 15–1. Schematic of the immune system.

CHAPTER 16

ANTIGEN PROCESSING

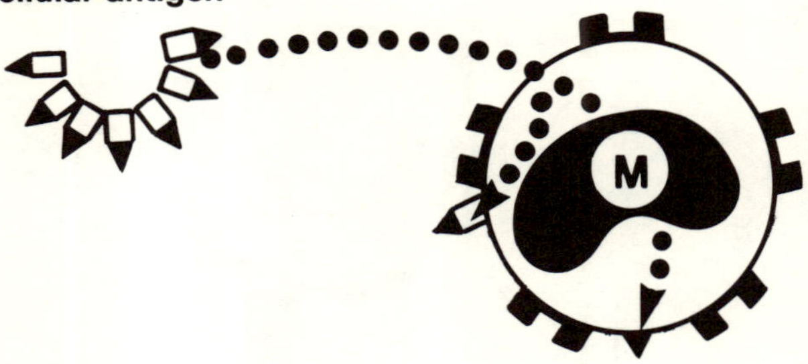

B-lymphocyte clones secrete immunoglobulin in response to an antigen introduced into the body. Similarly, T-lymphocyte clones respond to antigen by the production of cell-mediated immunity. T lymphocytes are found throughout the lymphoid system, but they cannot respond to an antigen until the antigen has first undergone an **antigen-processing step**. Only after the antigen is processed will the T-lymphocyte clones recognize and respond to that antigen (described in Chapter 17). Only after the antigen-specific T-lymphocyte clones are activated will B-lymphocyte clone activation proceed. It is thought that the mononuclear phagocyte and a few related cell types must first ingest the antigen and then somehow process it within its cytoplasm.

Mononuclear phagocytes appear to have a natural ability to recognize normal, healthy, self cells from dead cells and nonself invader cells. Mononuclear phagocytes are known to have a natural tendency to ingest dead cells and any nonself invader cells that are encountered. In order to activate T-lymphocyte clones, the antigens found on the ingested invader cells must be chemically modified (an enzyme-mediated reaction). The mononuclear phagocyte then reexpresses the processed antigen on its surface along with a unique set of membrane proteins known as **DR**, as shown in Figure 16–1 (DR proteins are discussed in Chapter 22). In Figure 16–1, the "native" (unprocessed) antigen from the nonself invader cell is processed by a mononuclear phagocyte and reexpressed on the mononuclear phagocyte membrane along with the DR proteins. This complex of *processed antigen* with DR will be the activation signal for the T lymphocytes. In addition, there is some native (unprocessed) antigen found on the mononuclear phagocyte membrane. This signal in combination with help from T lymphocytes activates the B lymphocytes.

Suggested Reading

Hood, L. E., I. L. Weissman, N. B. Wood, and J. H. Wilson. *Immunology*. Menlo Park, CA: Benjamin/Cummings, 1984.

Unanue, E. R. and A. S. Rosenthal (eds.). *Machrophage Regulation of Immunity*. New York: Academic Press, 1980.

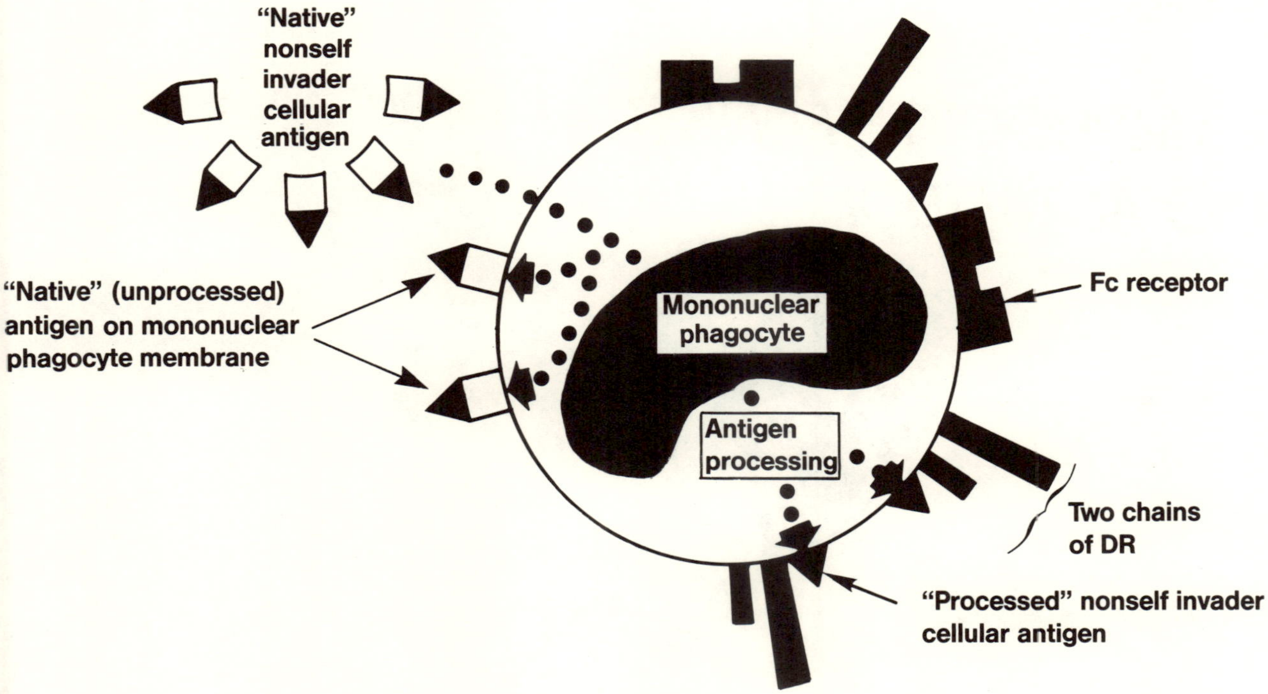

Figure 16–1. Details of antigen processing.

REVIEW QUESTIONS for Antigen Processing

1. What cell is principally responsible for antigen processing?

The mononuclear phagocyte is principally responsible for antigen processing. [p. 98]

2. What is meant by antigen processing?

Antigen processing means that an antigen must be ingested and enzymatically modified by a mononuclear phagocyte before it can initiate an immune response. [p. 98]

3. How does the antigen-processing event take place in the mononuclear phagocyte?

The mononuclear phagocyte must first ingest the antigen, process it (chemically modify it), and then reexpress it on its surface along with the two protein chains of DR. [p. 98]

CHAPTER 17

T-LYMPHOCYTE FUNCTION AND ACTIVATION

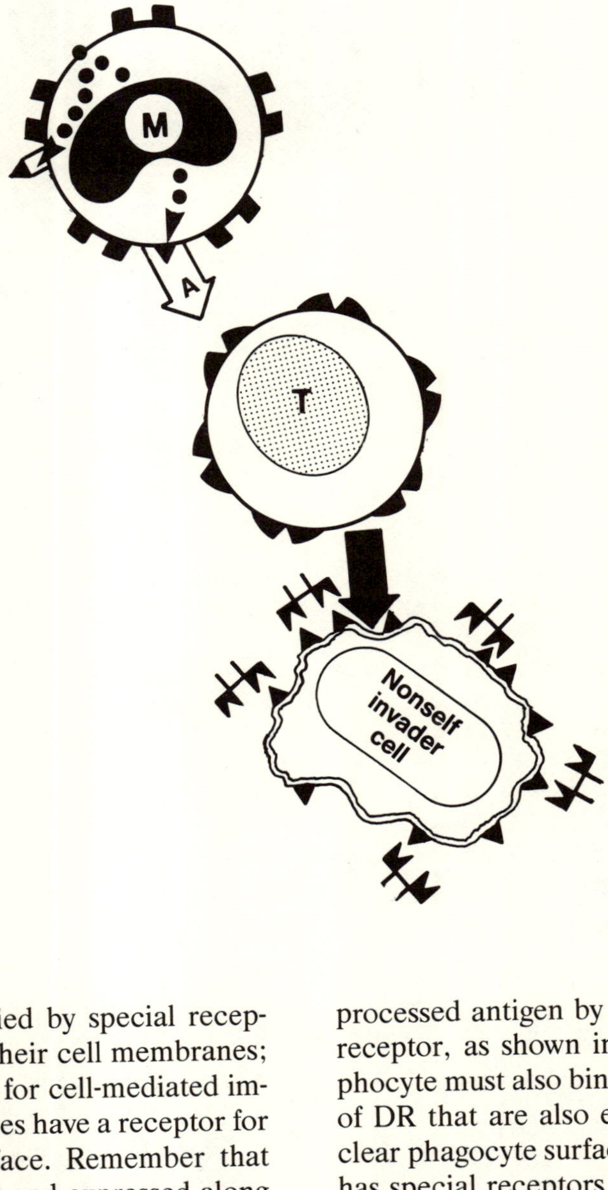

T-lymphocytes are identified by special receptors for antigen found on their cell membranes; these cells are responsible for cell-mediated immunity. T-lymphocyte clones have a receptor for antigen on their cell surface. Remember that antigen must be processed and expressed along with the DR molecule on the surface of the mononuclear phagocyte. The code for T-lymphocyte activation is somewhat complicated because T lymphocytes require at least two signals for activation to occur. In addition to binding processed antigen by the T-lymphocyte antigen receptor, as shown in Figure 17–1, the T lymphocyte must also bind to the two protein chains of DR that are also expressed on the mononuclear phagocyte surface. The T lymphocyte also has special receptors for this purpose. Thus, to be activated, the T lymphocyte requires both signals to be present at the same time. The concept of a lock and key can be used to visualize this stimulatory mechanism. If the T-lymphocyte receptors (for antigen and DR) and the

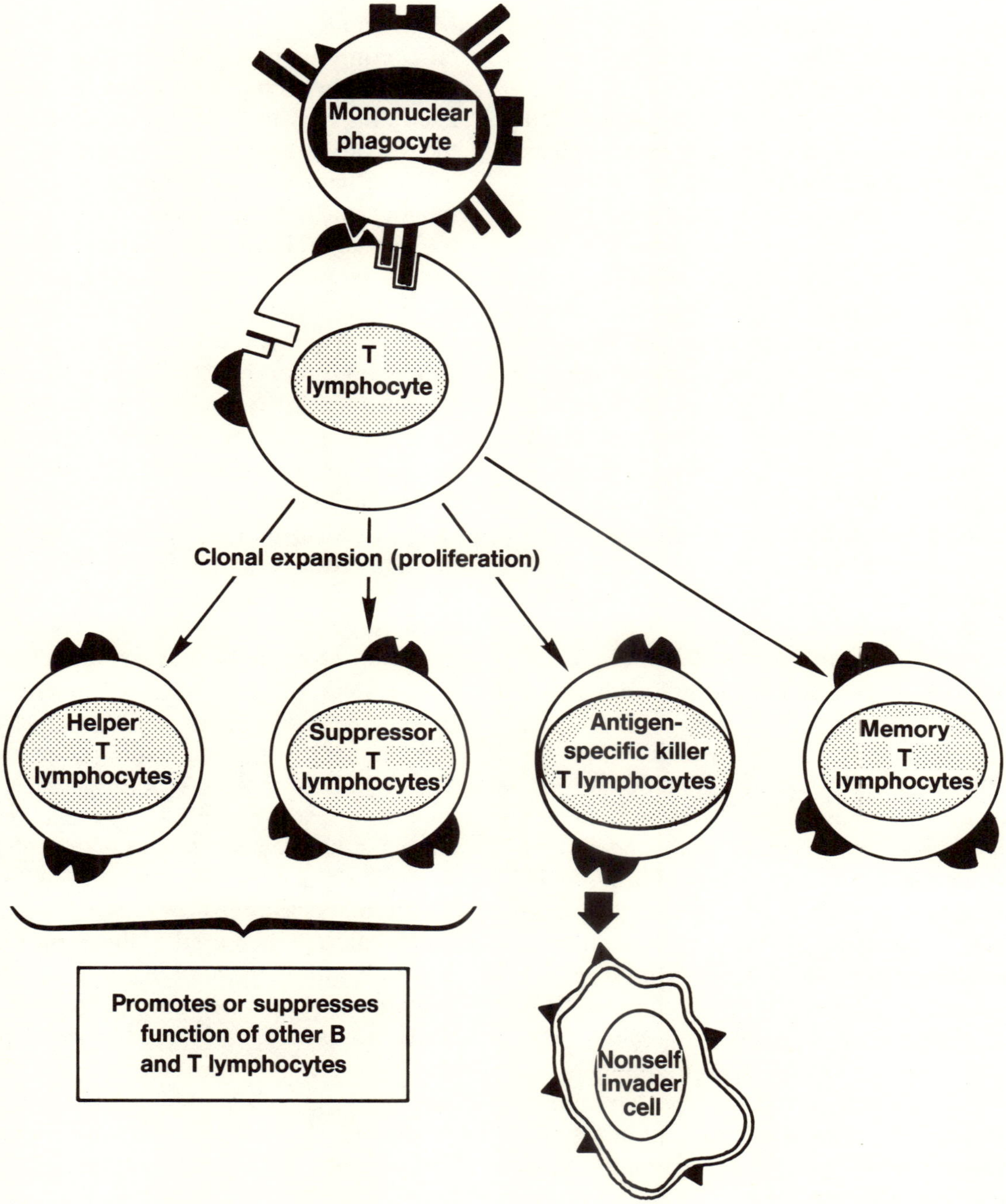

Figure 17–1. Details of T-lymphocyte activation.

surface molecules on the mononuclear phagocyte (processed antigen and DR) do not match exactly, then no T-lymphocyte activation will occur. Detailed information about DR is presented in Chapter 22.

Figure 17–1 shows a T lymphocyte receiving activation signals from a mononuclear phagocyte that bears the exact processed antigen to which this particular T lymphocyte is specific, plus the two protein chains of DR that complete the lock and key concept. The T lymphocyte, having been activated, begins clonal expansion (proliferation) into four distinct subsets of T lymphocytes.

The four T-lymphocyte subsets are 1) **helper** T lymphocytes, 2) **suppressor** T lymphocytes, 3) **antigen-specific killer** T lymphocytes, and 4) **memory** T lymphocytes.

Helper T lymphocytes stimulate enhanced function in other lymphocytes and mononuclear phagocytes; suppressor T lymphocytes are capable of dampening the same functions. In the overall schematic in Figure 15–1, you will notice dotted lines with a circled "m" (---m---) going from T lymphocytes to B lymphocytes, natural killer lymphocytes, and mononuclear phagocytes. The "m" stands for *modulation* (help or suppression), and the modulatory influences that T lymphocytes exert on the function of other cells is performed via helper or suppressor T lymphocytes. The overall function of the cell that is being influenced will reflect the overall balance between helper and/or suppressor T-lymphocyte influences. As you will see in the next chapter (on B-Lymphocyte activation) and in Chapter 24, the production of helper T lymphocytes is a critical step required for immunoglobulin (Ig) secretion.

The T-lymphocyte killer cell subset can directly kill target cells bearing a specific antigen, such as the nonself invader cell shown in Figure 17–1, although scientists do not fully understand the mechanism involved. This T-lymphocyte killer function is highly *antigen-specific* compared with other types of killing cells like mononuclear phagocytes, which are very *nonspecific* in the target cell types that they can kill. The killer T lymphocyte is capable of killing only those cells coated with the specific antigen (or closely related antigen) that the particular T-lymphocyte clone responds to, and not those nonself invader cells bearing any other antigen(s).

In the process of immunization, as discussed in Chapter 13, memory T lymphocytes, much like the B-lymphocyte memory clones, are also produced following activation of a T-lymphocyte clone. These cells provide memory for antigen-specific cell-mediated immune responses. Following clonal proliferation to a specific antigen, T-lymphocyte memory cells are established. Cell-mediated immune responses now can occur more rapidly following secondary exposure to the antigen because clonal expansion occurs much more rapidly.

T lymphocytes are responsible for the specific component of *cell-mediated immunity*. Within a few days of nonself invasion (with bacteria, fungi, viruses, and possibly tumor cells), the T lymphocytes of an immunized individual will surround the nonself invader and begin arranging for its destruction *directly* (via antigen-specific killer T lymphocytes) and *indirectly* (via the recruitment of nonspecific killer cells—mononuclear phagocytes, PMN, and NK lymphocytes). T lymphocytes must be able to communicate with other cells in order to coordinate the various cell types that can attack the antigen. T lymphocytes secrete a variety of signal polypeptides that travel to other cells and signal these cells to perform specific functions. Peptides (polypeptides) that are released from one cell and direct the function of other cells are a type of hormone known in immunology as **biological response modifiers (BRM)**. The BRM that are known to be made by T lymphocytes are called **lymphokines**. Lymphokines, and other BRM, will be discussed in a separate chapter, but note that these *signal peptides* have very potent effects on the overall immune responses. Examples of lymphokines include: 1) **gamma interferon (IFN_γ)**, which causes mononuclear phagocytes to have enhanced killing function; 2) **interleukin 2**, which acts as a *growth factor* for T lymphocytes, causing increased cellular proliferation; 3) **B-cell growth factor (BCGF)**, which causes B-lymphocyte clones to proliferate; and 4) **lymphotoxin (LT)**, which is secreted predominantly by killer T lymphocytes and can cause tumor target cell death. Certain helper and suppressor T lymphocytes work by secreting lymphokines (BRM) that are capable of modulating the function of responder cells; this function is discussed in greater detail in subsequent chapters.

Suggested Reading

Barrett, J. *Textbook of Immunology*. St. Louis, MO: Mosby, 1983.

Stites, D. P., J. D. Stobo, H. H. Fudenberg, and J. V. Wells. *Basic and Clinical Immunology,* 4th ed. Los Altos, CA: Lange Medical Publications, 1982.

REVIEW QUESTIONS for T-Lymphocyte Function and Activation

1. What is a T lymphocyte?

The T lymphocyte is responsible for the initiation of the specific component of cell-mediated immunity. It is a lymphocyte that bears antigen-specific receptors on its surface. [p. 100]

2. What two signals are required for activation of T lymphocytes?

The T-lymphocyte antigen and DR receptors must match exactly with both the processed antigen and the DR chains that are expressed on the mononuclear phagocyte's cell membrane. [p. 100]

3. What four subsets of T lymphocytes are made once the T lymphocyte is activated?

1) Helper T lymphocytes
2) Suppressor T lymphocytes
3) Antigen-specific killer T lymphocytes
4) Memory T lymphocytes

[p. 102]

4. What is the function of helper T lymphocytes?

Helper T lymphocytes stimulate enhanced immunologic function in other cells. [p. 102]

5. What is the function of suppressor T lymphocytes?

Suppressor T lymphocytes serve as controls to dampen immunologic responses of other cells. [p. 102]

6. What is the function of a killer T lymphocyte?

A killer T lymphocyte is antigen-specific and will only kill those targets that bear the antigen for which the killer cell has a receptor. [p. 102]

7. What is the function of memory T lymphocytes?

Memory T lymphocytes provide memory for the cell-mediated component of the immune response. [p. 102]

8. What are lymphokines?

Lymphokines are biological response modifiers (BRM) (signal peptide hormones), secreted by T lymphocytes, which are capable of directing the function of other cells in the area where nonself invasion is occurring. [p. 102]

9. Name four major lymphokines secreted by T lymphocytes.

1) IFN_{γ}—Gamma interferon
2) BCGF—B-cell growth factor
3) LT—Lymphotoxin
4) IL2—Interleukin 2

[p. 102]

10. What are some functions of these four lymphokines?

1) IFN_{γ}—causes enhanced killing function by mononuclear phagocytes.
2) BCGF—promotes B lymphocyte proliferation.
3) LT—lymphotoxin; causes tumor target cell death.
4) IL2—causes proliferation of other T lymphocytes.

[p. 102]

CHAPTER 18

B-LYMPHOCYTE ACTIVATION

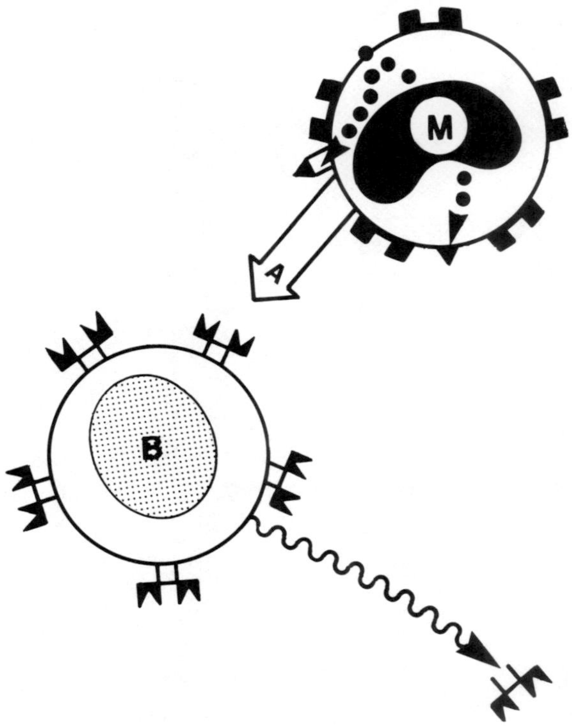

B lymphocytes are identified by surface immunoglobulin (sIg) found on their cell membranes; these cells are responsible for immunoglobulin (Ig) production. When does a B lymphocyte become activated to begin Ig production? Remember, like the T lymphocyte that has special receptors for processed antigen and DR, B lymphocytes also bear special receptors (sIg) for native (unprocessed) antigen on its outer membrane. This sIg is specific for one type of antigen, and therefore the B lymphocyte has an antigen-specific receptor on its surface (sIg) that will bind the native (unprocessed) antigen that is presented on the surface of the mononuclear phagocyte. Thus, B lymphocytes, which tend to be fixed in the lymphoid organs of the body, wait until they are exposed to that particular antigen (or a very closely related molecule) for which they are specific. As shown in Figure 18–1, the antigen on the mononuclear phagocyte surface is then recognized by the appropriate B-lymphocyte clone when it is bound to the B-lymphocyte sIg. The B lymphocyte then forms a sIg-antigen "cap" (these molecules move to a specific area on the surface of the cell). This is a certain sign of B-lymphocyte activation. Later, the cap is internalized by the cell. After ingesting this antigen-sIg cap and receiving a helper signal (B-cell growth factor [BCGF]) from helper T lymphocytes, two types of B lymphocytes can

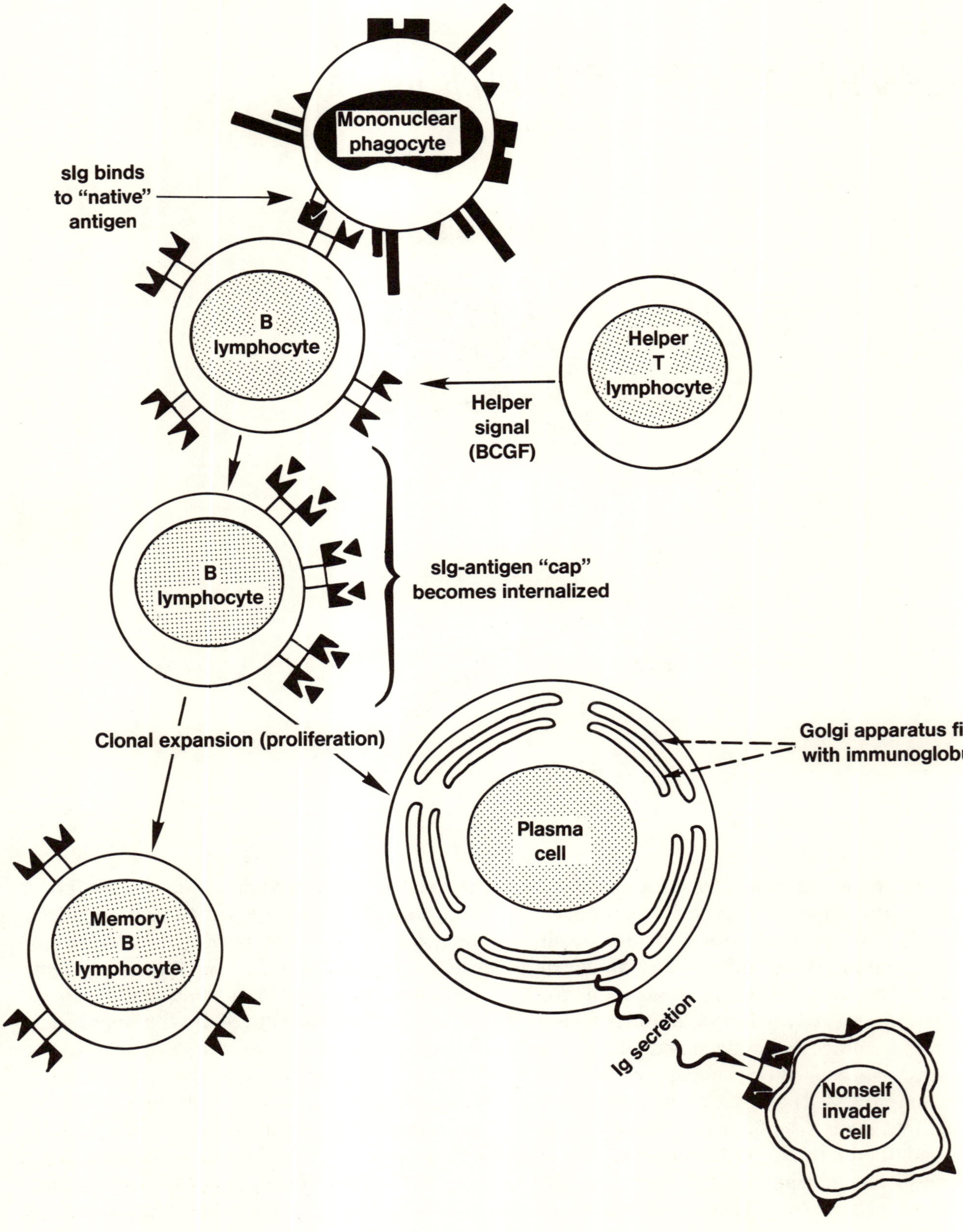

Figure 18–1. Details of B-lymphocyte activation.

be found to be **proliferating** (a limited expansion of cell numbers). One type of proliferating B lymphocyte loses its sIg entirely and instead becomes an Ig-secreting "factory" with large amounts of Ig found in its ribosomes and Golgi apparatus. This cell is known as a **plasma cell** and is the principal cell responsible for Ig secretion. The plasma cell clones do not express sIg, unlike the original B lymphocyte, but they do secrete immunoglobulin of the same idiotype (antigen-binding fragment as found on the sIg of the original B-lymphocyte clone). The second type of proliferating B lymphocyte is the **memory B lymphocyte**. The memory B lymphocyte is responsible for the recall component of the system, which is the basis for immunization.

Thus, if a person has been exposed to a specific bacterial antigen, such as the cell walls of the tetanus bacterium (tetanus toxoid), via primary immunization, the appropriate B lymphocyte clone will respond by binding to the native (unprocessed) antigen found on the membrane of the mononuclear phagocyte. After receiving a helper T lymphocyte signal (BCGF), the B-lymphocyte clone then proliferates and produces plasma cells that secrete tetanus toxoid-specific Ig. These Ig are released into the blood to seek and to bind with antigen throughout the body. The principal class of immunoglobulin secreted following this initial exposure to the tetanus antigen is **IgM**; 1–3 weeks elapse before significant amounts of IgM reactive with tetanus toxoid are found in the bloodstream. In addition, memory B lymphocytes for the antigen are created and will last for many years in the body. The entire process of B-lymphocyte activation and proliferation in response to a new antigen takes about 1–3 weeks. After the initial exposure, however, the system is primed; that is, B-lymphocyte memory has been established for tetanus antigen, and the next time tetanus toxoid is introduced, it is recognized and responded to within 1–3 days via the memory B lymphocytes. The antigen-binding fragment (idiotype) of the Ig secreted following secondary exposure to tetanus antigen is the same as following primary exposure. However, the secreted immunoglobulin will be of the *IgG* class, not the IgM class.

Suggested Reading

Barrett, J. T. *Textbook of Immunology*. St. Louis, MO: Mosby, 1983.

Hood, L. E., I. L. Weissman, W. B. Wood, and J. H. Wilson. *Immunology*. Menlo Park, CA: Benjamin/Cummings, 1984.

REVIEW QUESTIONS for B-Lymphocyte Activation

1. What is the definition of a B lymphocyte?

A B lymphocyte is a lymphocyte that bears surface Ig (sIg) on its cell membrane and upon activation will secrete Ig (via plasma cells). [p. 105]

2. What are the two steps required for B-lymphocyte activation?

Capping of the sIg-antigen complexes, and exposure to B-cell growth factor (BCGF) from helper T lymphocytes will cause B-lymphocyte proliferation (expansion of cells in number by division). [p. 105]

3. What are the two types of cells that result from the activation of a B-lymphocyte clone?

Plasma cells (Ig-secreting cells) and memory B lymphocytes result from activation of a B-lymphocyte clone. [p. 107]

4. What class of Ig is made upon primary exposure to an antigen? How long does this process take?

IgM is the class of Ig secreted following initial exposure to an antigen; the process takes 1–3 weeks. [p. 107]

5. What class of Ig is made following secondary exposure to an antigen? How long does this process take?

IgG is the class of Ig secreted following repeated exposure to an antigen; this process takes 1–3 days. [p. 107]

CHAPTER 19

THE COMPLEMENT COMPONENTS

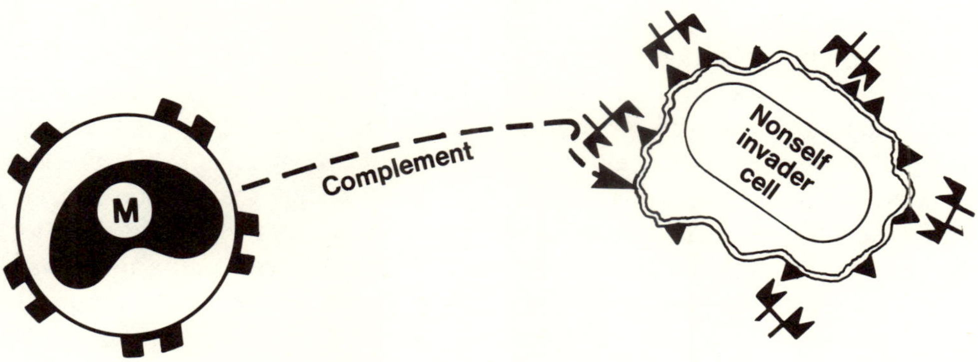

Recall that the complement system is the nonspecific component of humoral immunity. The **complement system (C)** consists of a series of proteins that circulate in an inactive form in the bloodstream. The complement system proteins can activate one another in a cascading sequence—in a stepwise action—like the different levels of a cascading waterfall. The complement components are principally synthesized by the mononuclear phagocytes. The majority of the C proteins are regulatory (rate-limiting) enzymes; however, the last five proteins in the C cascade perform an **effector function**. These five proteins are responsible for the ultimate destruction of the antigen.

The C proteins principally discussed in this chapter are those numbered C1 through C9. Of these, the five final effector proteins—C5, C6, C7, C8, and C9—are responsible for antigen destruction. The best way to visualize these last five proteins and their function is to view them as a **trochar**, a hollow, needle-like tube that is used in the practice of medicine to withdraw fluid. These proteins, when activated, form a trochar-like configuration that will attack any cell in the vicinity by poking a hole in its lipid bilayer (cell membrane) and allowing the intracellular matter to leak out, thus killing the cell. Figure 19–1 demonstrates a highly simplified picture of the C system.

The C components are short polypeptide enzymes each of which is completely inactive until it is activated by the enzyme above it in the cascade. At this time, it becomes activated and is able to activate the next enzyme in the sequence of the cascade. To initiate the C cascade, C1, the first enzyme in the cascade must become activated. *The major C-activating signal occurs when IgM or IgG molecules become associated with antigen.* When IgM or IgG binds antigen, a conformational change occurs along the entire Ig molecule. This change exposes a special C1 binding and activation site in the Fc constant region (close to the hinge region) of the Ig molecule. C1 in its inactive form is denoted as C1 and, when activated, is denoted as $C\bar{1}$. The sequence of events that follows activation of C1 by the IgM or IgG enzymatic mechanism is called the **classical complement activation pathway**. When C1 becomes $C\bar{1}$, it activates C4 and C2 to form a second functional enzyme unit called $C\overline{4,2}$. (Note that the activation of the C components does not always follow their numerical sequence.) The activated enzyme C$\overline{4,2}$ causes C3 to become activated. When the C3 molecule becomes activated by C$\overline{4,2}$, it becomes the active complement component, named C$\overline{3}$. C$\overline{3}$ is the active form of C3, and it acts upon the next complement component C5, which when activated becomes C$\overline{5}$. C$\overline{5}$ then triggers the assembly of the **membrane attach complex** (the trochar).

In the presence of C$\overline{5}$, the inactive molecules C6, C7, C8, and C9 come together to form the membrane attack complex—C$\overline{5,6,7,8,9}$—a trochar capable of poking holes in cell membranes. Remember, complement is a nonspecific destroyer of cellular antigens. It does not have any specificity; thus, *any* cells located in the area where the C system has been activated, whether they are self or nonself, will be destroyed—*lysed*. The C attack complexes will be found where the greatest concentration of C is being activated, which, of course, is where the IgM or IgG is bound to an antigen. Thus, Ig is the only directing factor that focuses the terminal complement attack units on target. There is simply a high concentration of the complement trochar units in an area where IgG or IgM is bound to antigen.

Besides the classical pathway there is an alternate pathway that will also activate C. This pathway is called the **alternate pathway** (shown in the diamond in Figure 19–1. The alternate pathway is very complicated and bypasses factors C1, C4, and C2 but merges with the classical pathway at the level of C3. The initiating factors for the alternate pathway, as opposed to antigen binding by IgG or IgM antibody as in the classical pathway, are biomolecules that are predominantly found in the cell walls of bacteria and yeast. Other factors like IgA and IgE, when aggregated (clumped together), can also activate this alternate complement activating system. The alternate pathway is a backup complement activating system that can be utilized when specific antibody (Ig) for an antigen is not available.

The alternate pathway activates C3 directly to generate the active enzyme C$\overline{3}$. The rest of the C activation is identical to what has previously been described. C$\overline{3}$ activates C5 to generate C$\overline{5}$, which then activates the C$\overline{5,6,7,8,9}$ membrane attack complex.

Suggested Reading

Eisen, H. M. *Immunology*. Hagerstown, MD: Harper & Row, 1980.

Hood, L. E., I. L. Weissman, W. B. Wood, and J. H. Wilson. *Immunology*. Menlo Park, CA: Benjamin/Cummings, 1984.

REVIEW QUESTIONS for The Complement Components

1. What is the overall function of complement in the immune response?

   Complement (C) is the nonspecific component of humoral immunity that allows IgG- or IgM-coated cells to be destroyed. [p. 109]

2. Where are the complement components synthesized?

   C components are principally synthesized by mononuclear phagocytes. [p. 109]

3. What are the names of the C components of the classical pathway?

   C1 through C9 are the C components of the classical pathway. [p. 109]

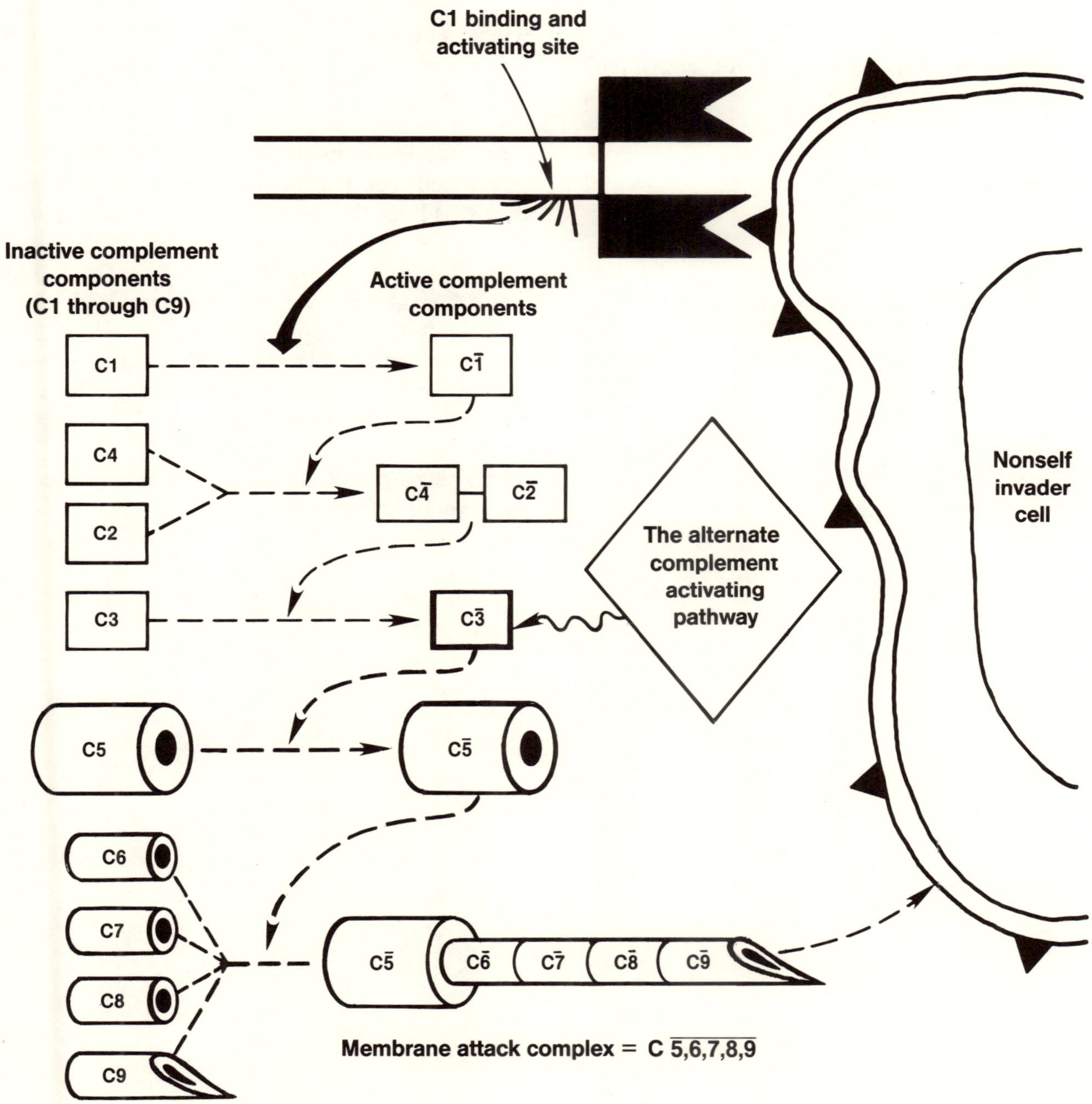

Figure 19–1. Details of the complement components.

4. How does C actually lyse a cell?	Upon final activation, the membrane attack complex ($C\overline{5,6,7,8,9}$) pokes a hole in the cell's membrane, allowing the cellular contents to leak out. [p. 110]
5. What is the function of the first four components of the classical pathway of C activation?	These components are enzymes that activate one another in a cascade fashion in the classical pathway of C activation. [p. 110]
6. What is the function of the last five components of the C cascade?	The last five components of the cascade, when assembled, become the membrane attack complex that lyses the cell by poking holes in its cell membrane. [p. 110]
7. What is the role of the alternate pathway?	The alternate pathway is an immunoglobulin-independent back-up mechanism by which the C system can be activated. It depends predominantly on biomolecules found on bacterial cell walls as the activation signal. [p. 110]
8. Where do the alternate and classical pathways merge?	The alternate and classical pathways merge at the level of C3. [p. 110]

CHAPTER 20

MONONUCLEAR PHAGOCYTE, POLYMORPHONUCLEAR GRANULOCYTE, AND NATURAL KILLER LYMPHOCYTE FUNCTION

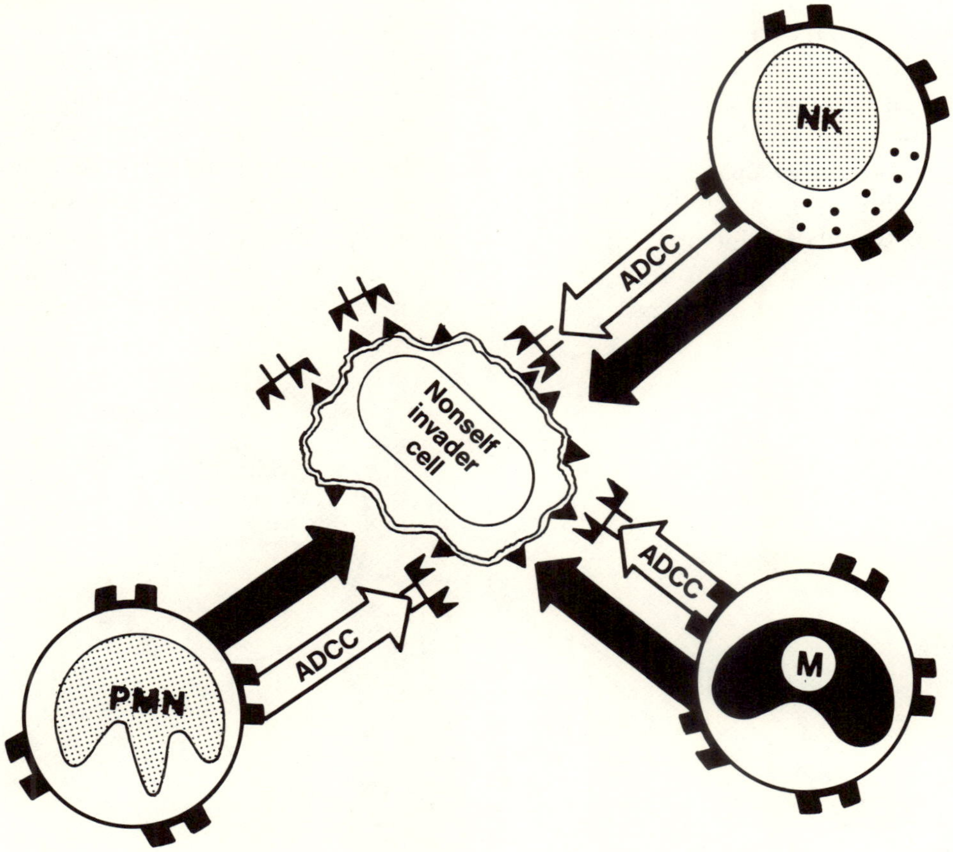

Mononuclear phagocytes, polymorphonuclear granulocytes (PMN), and natural killer (NK) lymphocytes are the nonspecific effector cells of the cell-mediated immune response. Mononuclear phagocytes, PMN, and NK lymphocytes are able to destroy a variety of targets, but they do this *nonspecifically*. In order for these cells to be targeted on any particular invader cell, they must be directed to do so by specific signals that will be discussed later.

Mononuclear phagocytes were introduced in Chapter 16. They are mobile cells capable of ingesting (phagocytizing) a wide range of targets. Mononuclear phagocytes exist in three forms in the body: **promonocytes**, **monocytes**, and **macrophages**. Promonocytes are the earliest differentiation step of the mononuclear phagocytes away from the common stem cell, as discussed in Chapter 12, and only exist in the bone marrow. When promonocytes mature into monocytes, which are cells with a characteristic horseshoe-shaped nucleus, they are ejected into the bloodstream. Within 48 hours, monocytes leave the bloodstream to become lodged in *lymphoid tissues* (the **reticuloendothelial system**—liver, spleen, and lymph nodes). Once in the reticuloendothelial tissues, monocytes differentiate into macrophages—"large eater" cells. In addition to antigen processing, mononuclear phagocytes appear capable of distinguishing live, normal self cells from dead self cells or invader cells (bacteria, fungi, and tumor cells). Mononuclear phagocytes also participate in the removal of dead self cells and live or dead invader cells. Like T lymphocytes that secrete biological response modifiers (BRM) called *lymphokines*, monocytes release a large number of important biological response modifiers (BRM), known as **monokines**. Examples include: 1) **alpha interferon** (**IFN**$_a$), which causes boosting of NK lymphocyte killing; 2) **colony stimulating factor (CSF)**, which causes proliferation of mononuclear phagocytes and PMN in the bone marrow; 3) **interleukin 1 (IL1)**, which stimulates T-lymphocyte proliferation; and 4) **tumor necrosis factor (TNF)**, which causes tumor cell death. (These monokines are discussed further in Chapter 24.)

The **PMN** (polymorphonuclear) granulocytes are mobile phagocytic cells that are short lived (they only live about 2 days in the bloodstream) and have a nucleus with many lobes. The major function of the PMN is to attack bacteria and fungus invaders of the body. The PMN are found mainly in the bloodstream and in body tissues infected by bacteria or fungi.

The *NK lymphocyte* seems to exist predominantly in one form: as a large, non-T, non-B lymphocyte with prominent granules in its cytoplasm. For this reason, NK lymphocytes are also referred to as **large granular lymphocytes (LGL)**. Large granular lymphocytes exist throughout the lymphoid system and are very abundant in the bloodstream. The main function of NK lymphocytes appears to be the destruction of tumor cell

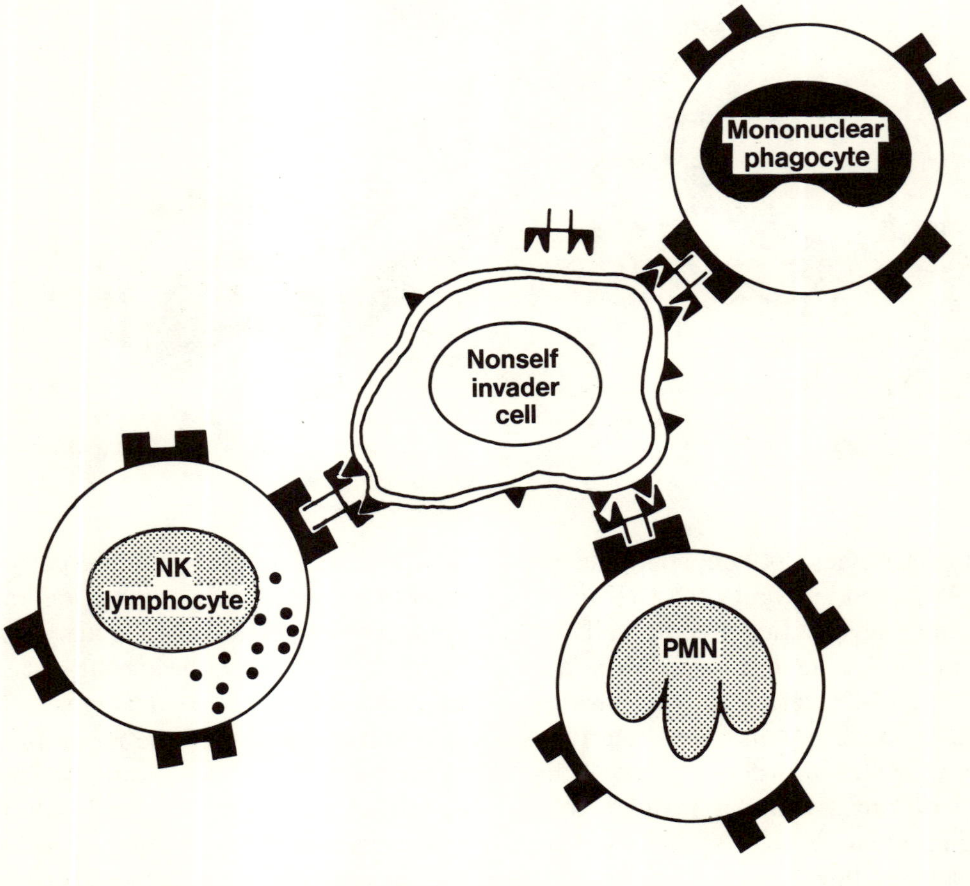

Figure 20–1. Details of antibody-dependent cellular cytotoxicity (ADCC).

targets and virus-infected cell targets.

Target cell killing (**cytotoxicity**) can be accomplished by two distinct mechanisms: one type of cytotoxicity requires immunoglobulin—**antibody-dependent cellular cytotoxicity (ADCC)**; the other type does not require antibody and is called **natural**, or **spontaneous**, **cytotoxicity**. As shown in Figure 20–1, ADCC occurs when a target cell (nonself invader cell in this figure) is coated with IgG antibody (immunoglobulin). This cell is now highly vulnerable to attack by any killer cell that bears receptors for the Fc portion of IgG antibody (Fc receptors) on its cell membrane. Mononuclear phagocytes, PMN, and NK lymphocytes bear Fc receptors in great abundance and are highly efficient target cell killers using the ADCC mechanism. Mononuclear phagocytes and PMN may ingest IgG-coated targets; NK lymphocytes, however, are not phagocytic. Obviously, because ADCC requires antibody (IgG), it is ultimately the B lymphocyte that directs the mononuclear phagocytes, PMN, and NK lymphocytes to the appropriate target by secreting the antibody that binds to the target cell. *Antibody alone will not harm a target cell.* ADCC or complement-mediated lysis (Chapter 19) must occur in order for the antibody-coated target cell to be killed.

ADCC is a highly efficient mechanism for killing nonself invader targets. If B lymphocytes have not released Ig yet, however, a back-up mechanism for defense exists. The second mechanism for target cell killing is *natural*, or *spontaneous*, cytotoxicity (Figure 20–2). *NK lymphocytes* kill a wide range of tumor cells and virally infected targets without antibody (in contrast to ADCC and in contrast to the antigen-specific target cell killing by killer T lymphocyte clones). The Fc receptors of NK lymphocytes are not involved in **natural killing**. Furthermore, natural killing can be boosted if NK lymphocytes are exposed to *alpha interferon* (IFN_{α})

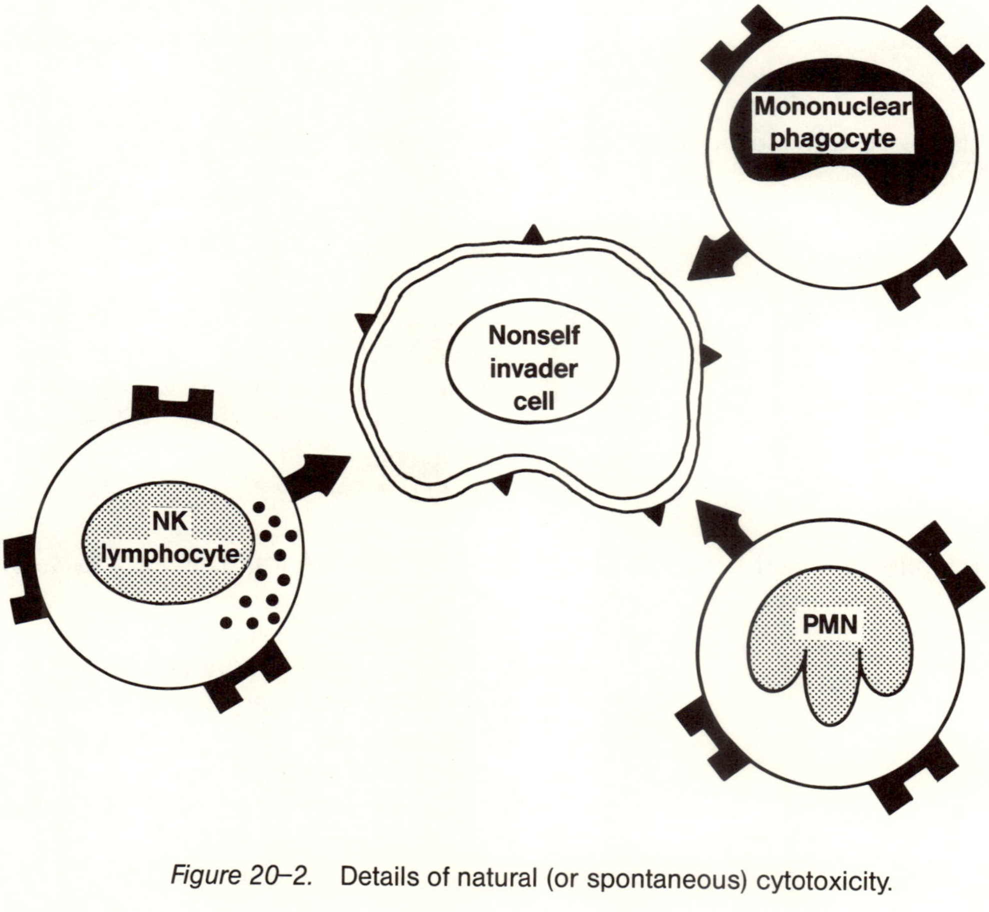

Figure 20–2. Details of natural (or spontaneous) cytotoxicity.

(made by mononuclear phagocytes) at the time that they encounter a target cell (Chapter 24).

In addition to participating in ADCC, PMN can kill certain nonself invader targets quite efficiently without the need for antibody to be coating the target cell. PMN are a first line of defense against bacterial and fungal infection and tend to kill these targets by ingesting them.

Mononuclear phagocytes are also capable of spontaneously eliminating target cells (bacteria, fungi, tumor cells, and dead normal cells) independent of the ADCC mechanism. The spontaneous killing of target cells by mononuclear phagocytes can be boosted by *gamma interferon* (IFN_γ). The bulk of cell-mediated immunity involves mononuclear phagocytes as follows: 1) antigen-specific T lymphocytes move into the area of target cell invasion; 2) they recruit mononuclear phagocytes into the area of invasion; and 3) by secreting IFN_γ, T lymphocytes activate the mononuclear phagocytes to kill the target cell (Chapter 24). Almost 80 percent of the cell-mediated immunity leukocytes surrounding a nonself invader are recruited mononuclear phagocytes; the remaining 20 percent are antigen-specific killer and helper T lymphocytes.

Suggested Reading

Barrett, J. T. *Textbook of Immunology*. St. Louis, MO: Mosby, 1983.

Eisen, H. N *Immunology*. Hagerstown, MD: Harper & Row, 1980.

REVIEW QUESTIONS for Mononuclear Phagocyte, Polymorphonuclear Granulocyte, AND Natural Killer Lymphocyte Function

1. What cells are responsible for the nonspecific component of the cell-mediated immune response?

Mononuclear phagocytes, polymorphonuclear granulocytes (PMN), and natural killer (NK) lymphocytes are responsible for the nonspecific component. [p. 113]

2. What are the three forms of mononuclear phagocytes?

1) Promonocytes
2) Monocytes
3) Macrophages

[p. 113]

3. Where are the three forms of mononuclear phagocytes located?

1) Promonocytes are found in the bone marrow.
2) Monocytes are found in the peripheral blood.
3) Macrophages are found in the reticuloendothelial system (liver, spleen, and lymph nodes).

[p. 113–114]

4. Name four monokines and describe their functions.

1) Alpha interferon (IFN_α)—boosts NK lymphocyte killing.
2) Colony stimulating factor (CSF)—causes proliferation of mononuclear phagocytes and PMN in the bone marrow.
3) Interleukin 1 (IL1)—stimulates the proliferation of T lymphocytes.
4) Tumor necrosis factor (TNF)—causes tumor cell death.

[p. 114]

5. What are the general characteristics of the PMN?	Most PMN are ameboid, phagocytic cells. They are short-lived (2 days) and have a multi-lobed nucleus. [p. 114]
6. Where are PMN found?	PMN are found in the bloodstream and in bacterial or fungal-infected tissues. [p. 114]
7. What are the characteristics of the natural killer (NK) lymphocytes?	The natural killer lymphocytes are non-T, non-B lymphocytes with large granules in their cytoplasm. They are also known as large granular lymphocytes (LGL). [p. 114]
8. Where are natural killer lymphocytes found?	Natural killer lymphocytes are found in lymphoid tissues and in the bloodstream. [p. 114]
9. What are the two forms of cytotoxicity?	1) Antibody-dependent cellular cytotoxicity (ADCC) 2) Natural or spontaneous killing [p. 115]
10. What is the mechanism of antibody-dependent cellular cytotoxicity (ADCC)?	After a target cell becomes coated with antibody (IgG immunoglobulin), any cell bearing Fc receptors can destroy it (mononuclear phagocytes, PMN, or NK lymphocytes). [p. 115]
11. Which cell directs the mononuclear phagocytes, PMN, and NK lymphocytes to kill a target cell by ADCC?	The B lymphocyte directs the killing of target cells by ADCC by releasing the appropriate IgG antibody (via plasma cells) which binds to the target cell. [p. 115]
12. What is spontaneous or natural killing?	Mononuclear phagocytes, PMN, and NK lymphocytes have a natural ability to destroy certain nonself invader cells. [p. 115]
13. Name the principal cellular targets of the NK lymphocyte.	Tumor cells and virally infected cells are the principal targets of the NK lymphocyte. [p. 115]
14. Name an agent that is capable of boosting the natural killing function of NK lymphocytes.	Alpha interferon (IFN_{α}) is a natural killing agent. [p. 115]
15. Name the principal cellular targets of the mononuclear phagocytes.	The principal targets are bacteria, viruses, fungi, tumor cells, and dead normal cells. [p. 116]
16. Name a BRM that can boost spontaneous killing by mononuclear phagocytes.	Gamma interferon (IFN_{γ}) can boost natural killing. [p. 116]
17. What are the principal cellular targets of the PMN?	The principal targets of PMN are bacteria and fungi. [p. 116]

CHAPTER 21

REVIEW OF SCHEMATIC DIAGRAM OF THE IMMUNE RESPONSE

In the last 5 chapters we reviewed the various components of the overall immune response. The schematic diagram of that process is presented once again in Figure 21–1 to reestablish the relationships among the various components. Figure 21–1 depicts the overall immune response to the antigens on a nonself invader cell. The mononuclear phagocytes appear to have an innate ability to distinguish self cells from invader cells; invader cells and dead self cells tend to be rapidly ingested. However, B- and T-lymphocyte clones cannot respond to the nonself invader antigens until they have been processed by the mononuclear phagocyte. Processed antigens are reexpressed on the mononuclear phagocyte membrane in association with the DR molecules. Some native (unprocessed) antigen is also found on the mononuclear phagocyte membrane to which the B lymphocyte can bind.

Antigen-specific T-lymphocyte clones (antigen-specific component of cell-mediated immunity) can be activated when the processed antigen is on the surface of the mononuclear phagocyte, but processed antigen must be in association with the appropriate DR molecules. Once they are activated, the T-lymphocyte clones proliferate (differentiate) into four subsets: *helper*, *suppressor*, *antigen-specific killer*, and *memory T lymphocytes*. Helper and suppressor T-lymphocyte subsets serve the function of figuratively turning other lymphocytes and mononuclear phagocytes on and off. Each antigen-specific killer T-lymphocyte clone can kill only one specific type of nonself invader cell. Memory T lymphocytes serve as a rapid recall mechanism to activate cell-mediated immunity during subsequent antigenic invasions. A major function of activated antigen-specific killer T lymphocytes is to recruit mononuclear phagocytes to the target area to aid in target cell destruction. A major mechanism whereby T lymphocytes communicate with other cell types is through the secretion of peptide signals known as *lymphokines*. Lymphokines (biological response modifiers [BRM]) secreted by T lymphocytes include gamma interferon (IFN_{γ}), interleukin 2 (IL2), B-cell growth factor (BCGF), and lymphotoxin (LT).

B-lymphocyte clones bind to the native (unprocessed) antigen found on the surface of mononuclear phagocytes, but they also *require* a helper signal (BCGF) from helper T lymphocytes in order to be activated. B lymphocytes then proliferate to become Ig-secreting plasma cells and memory B lymphocytes. The secreted Ig then binds to the antigens found on the nonself invader cell (antigen-specific component of humoral immunity). Ig alone cannot kill the tumor cell; either complement (nonspecific component of humoral immunity) or an Fc receptor-bearing killer cell (nonspecific component of cell-mediated immunity) is required. Mononuclear phagocytes provide both of these functions; they secrete the complement components that are activated by the immunoglobulin–antigen complex and poke holes in the tumor cells. Mononuclear phagocytes also bind to IgG antibody-coated tumor target cells and kill them; this function is called antibody-dependent cellular cytotoxicity (ADCC). Natural killer (NK) lymphocytes and PMN are also capable of ADCC.

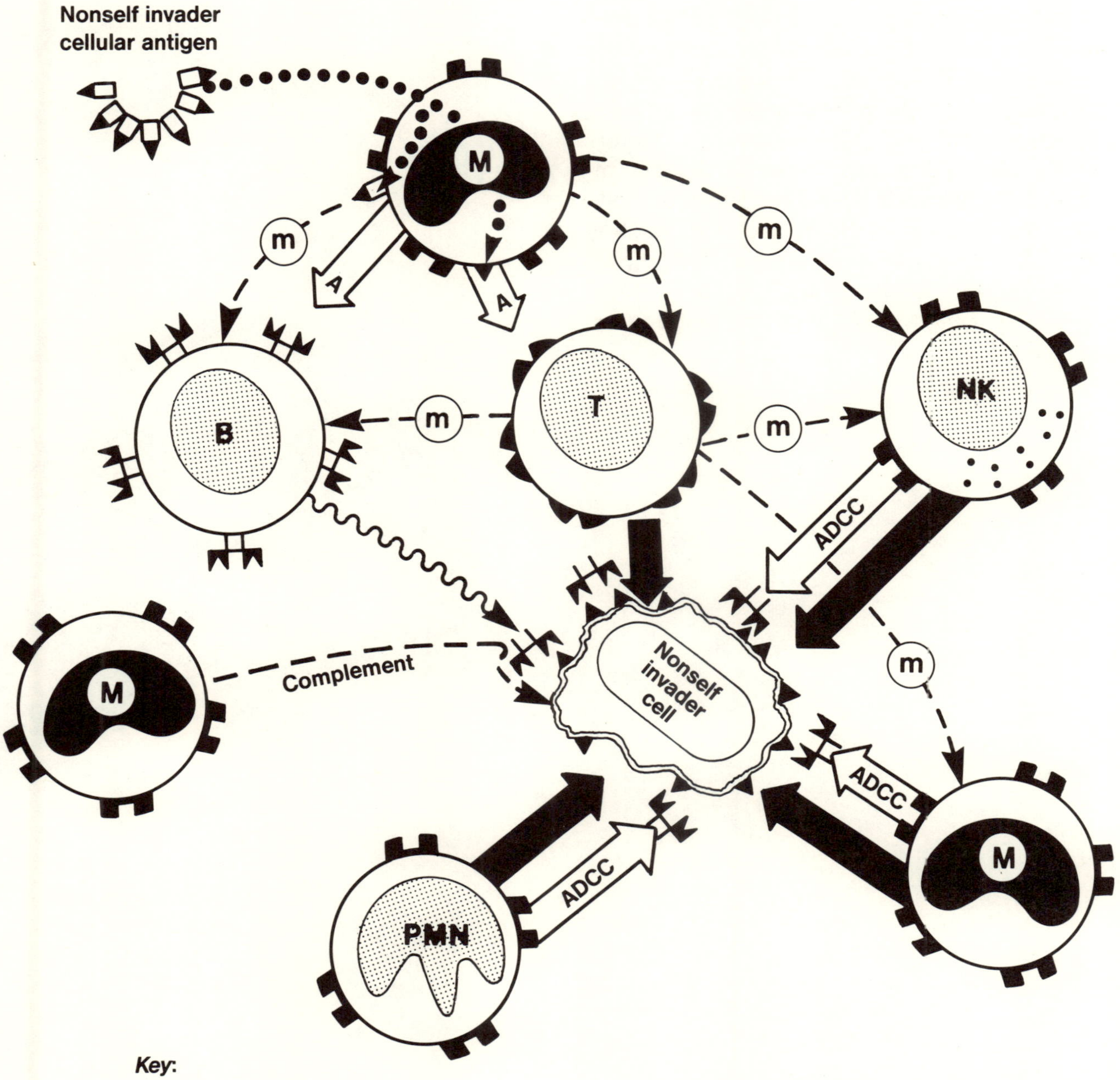

Key:

A = Activation	(m) = Modulation (help or suppression or both)
ADCC = Antibody-dependent cellular cytotoxicity	M = Mononuclear phagocyte
••• = Antigen processing	NK = NK lymphocyte
B = B lymphocyte	= Nonself invader antigen receptors on T cells
= Direct nonself invader cell killing	= Nonself invader antigen specific immunoglobulin
= Immunoglobulin Fc receptors	PMN = Polymorphonuclear granulocytes
= Immunoglobulin release	T = T Lymphocyte

Figure 21–1. Schematic of the immune system.

Mononuclear phagocytes, PMN, and NK lymphocytes represent the nonspecific component of cell-mediated immunity. They can kill a wide range of target cells spontaneously, or by antibody-dependent (ADCC) mechanisms. Mononuclear phagocytes also release a number of potent BRM (monokines) that influence, or modulate, the function of B, T, and NK lymphocytes. Representative monokines include alpha interferon (IFN_a), interleukin 1, (IL1), colony stimulating factor (CSF), and tumor necrosis factor (TNF).

CHAPTER 22

HUMAN LEUKOCYTE ANTIGENS (HLA)

Much of our understanding of the human leukocyte antigen (HLA) system is derived from immunological research studies originally performed with mice. Investigators found that mice with the same genetic make-up (same strain) behaved the same immunologically. That is to say, if two mice of a given strain were innoculated with the same antigen, both mice would respond immunologically in exactly the same fashion. For example, two mice of the same strain would produce similar amounts of IgG in response to the same antigen. In addition, mice of the same strain would *accept* organ grafts (transplantation) from one another; mice of different strains would *reject* organ grafts from one another. The mouse genes (called H–2 genes) that control these immunologic functions are located in a region on chromosome #17 in mice, known as the **major histocompatibility complex (MHC)**. The detection of genes that control immunologic responses in animals (H–2) promoted the search for MHC genes in humans. Human Leukocyte Antigen genes or **HLA** genes are a series of genes, in the HLA system found on the human chromosome #6, that code for proteins. HLA genes are expressed on most cells of the body, including the cells of the immune system. They correlate with the specific types of immune responses that human leukocytes can carry out. (Note that this chapter deals with the genetics of the HLA system, and it may be helpful to review Chapter 11 before proceeding.)

The infinite variety of immune responses is sometimes linked to the expression of certain HLA protein antigens on the surface of leukocytes. Persons who bear a certain HLA protein on their leukocytes (actually, these proteins are found on most cells of the body) are very likely to express an associated type of immune response. The mechanisms for the association between HLA proteins and immune responses are not well understood, but it is recognized that the types of HLA protein antigens on an individual's leukocytes are the primary factors in detemining whether or not foreign tissue grafts will be accepted or rejected. It might be a good idea to take a moment to clarify the use of the word *antigen* in the context of HLA. *Antigens* are nonself molecules. The HLA proteins (antigens) on an individual's leukocytes are, however, the mechanism by which self is determined. The HLA self proteins found on one individual's cells will become the principal nonself HLA *antigens* recognized when those cells are injected into another individual. The HLA proteins (antigens) found on the surface of your cells are not considered antigens when they are inside your body; they are part of self.

HLA antigens are actually identified in the laboratory by mixing the leukocytes of one individual with the serum (cell-free liquid portion of the blood) of another individual in a test tube to see whether they are compatible. If they are incompatible, the HLA antigens from one individual's leukocytes are perceived as *antigens* by the immunoglobulins found in the incompatible serum. An understanding of HLA typing is important because the leukocytes of each individual bear a unique HLA antigen code. Knowledge of this HLA code may allow prediction of which immunologic diseases each individual is susceptible to, or which tissue types can be transplanted into any given person. Knowledge of the HLA system will also help you understand the importance of HLA antigens in the activation of T lymphocytes by mononuclear phagocytes.

Let us review the six basic points of genetics; they must be clearly understood to comprehend the HLA system:

1) For every protein made in the body, there are two corresponding gene sites, one on each of the matching chromosomes at the gene site that contains the DNA code for the desired protein.
2) More than one gene (alleles) coding for different, variant (abnormal or less common) proteins may exist in the population for any given gene site.
3) Only two alleles for any given gene site can be inherited by any one individual (or each cell of that individual).
4) Two normal (most common) genes will code for a genotypically and phenotypically normal cell.
5) Two identical variant alleles will code for a genotypically and phenotypically abnormal cell.
6) If a cell has one normal and one variant allele, the cell will be genotypically abnormal, but the phenotype (function) depends on whether the variant allele codes for a dominant, recessive or coexpressive trait.

In the HLA system, every gene site is known to have multiple alleles; they are all coexpressed. There is no one normal (most common) gene for any of the HLA system proteins; just a large pool of alleles each coding for slightly different variants of the protein coded for at each gene site. From the multiple alleles that can occupy each HLA gene site, any given individual (and the cells of that individual) can only inherit two. If a cell inherits two different alleles at a given HLA gene site, *two* slightly different HLA proteins will be *coexpressed* on the surface of the cell.

There are three different general classes of HLA genes: **classes (HLA) I, II, and III**. These three classes of genes are found bunched tightly together on chromosome #6 of humans. *Class I* HLA genes code for cell surface proteins acting as recognition molecules that are identified by killer-T lymphocytes (discussed below). *Class II* HLA genes code for cell surface proteins involved in the cooperation and interaction between cells of the immune system (discussed below). *Class III* HLA genes code for several different types of proteins. The most studied class III gene products are certain of the *complement components* (reviewed in Chapter 19).

The *class I* HLA genes code for three distinct types of proteins called **HLA-A**, **HLA-B**, and **HLA-C**. These three proteins are found on most cells in the body, except red blood cells. To date, immunologists have discovered approximately 23 alleles at the HLA-A gene site (other alleles are suspected), 48 alleles at the HLA-B gene site, and 8 alleles at the HLA-C gene site. Although there are numerous possible alleles that can occupy each gene site, remember that any given cell can possess only two alleles at one time. Both of the proteins that the two alleles code for are coexpressed on the cell surface. However, as shown in Figure 22–1, the HLA-A, -B, and -C proteins are coexpressed on the surface of the cell only if they are associated with a small protein known as **beta two (β_2) microglobulin**. The gene that codes for the β_2 microglobulin protein is not found on chromosome #6 but on chromosome #15. When the cell assembles its HLA proteins (A, B, and C), these proteins accumulate in the cytoplasm but are not expressed on the cell surface until β_2 microglobulin is manufactured and is physically associated with the HLA antigens. Only then can both proteins be expressed on the cell surface together.

To summarize: 1) HLA-A, -B, and -C protein antigens are determined by DNA codes found in three gene sites (loci) on chromosome #6. 2) These three loci are called the HLA-A, HLA-B, and HLA-C gene sites. There are multiple alleles for each gene site. 3) The two alleles for each HLA gene that a given cell inherits are both transcribed and translated into proteins that are coexpressed on the surface of the cell in association with the protein, β_2 microglobulin. Thus, every leukocyte will have expressed on its surface 1) two HLA-A proteins, 2) two HLA-B proteins, and 3) two HLA-C proteins. The two HLA-A proteins could be the *same* (**homozygous**)

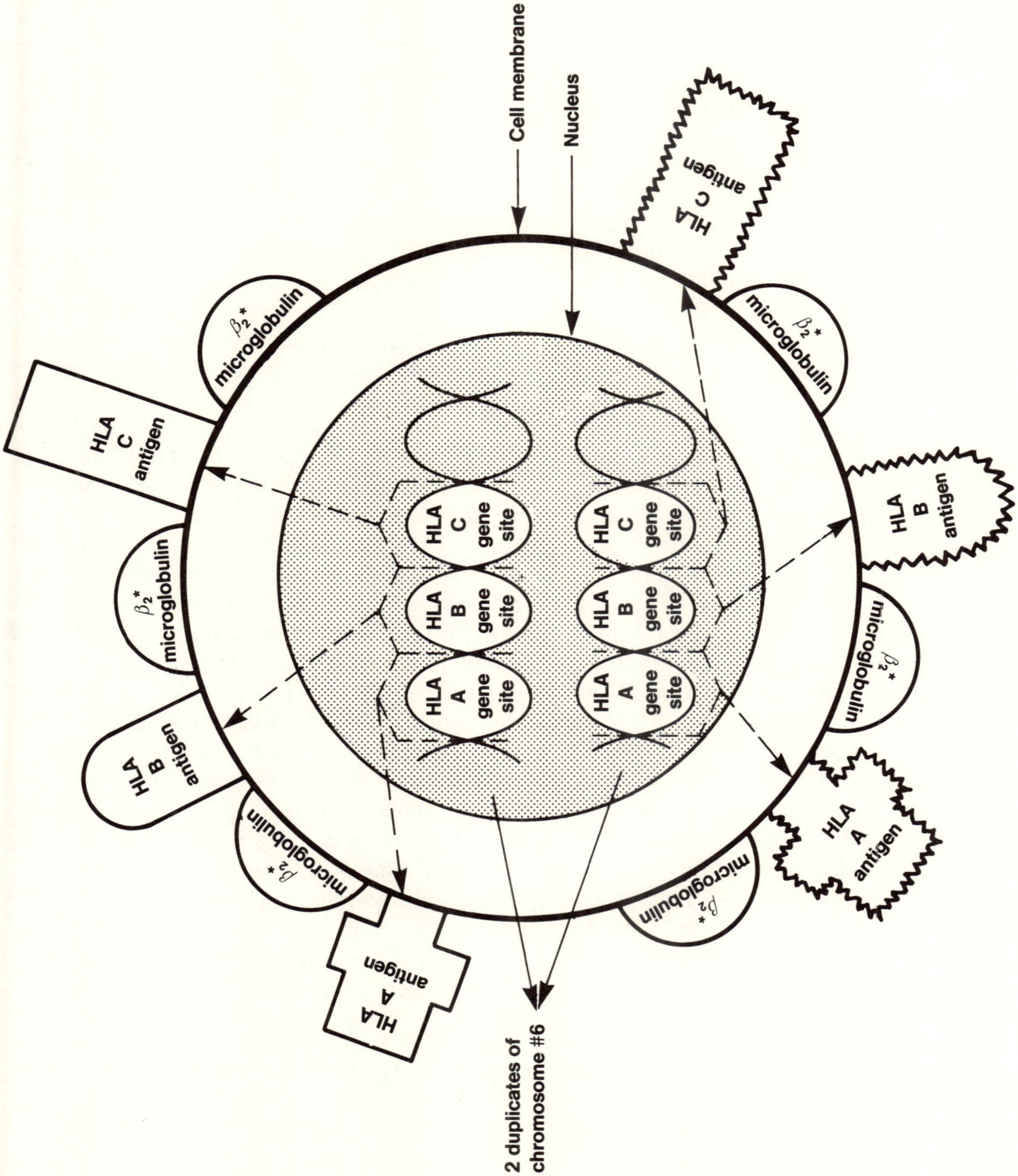

Figure 22–1. Genetic basis for HLA antigen expression.

or, much more likely, they could be *different*, from two different coexpressed alleles (**heterozygous**) (as shown in Figure 22–1). The number of different *self-codes* that can be generated by such a system is astronomical. In fact, the statistical chance of any two random individuals having exactly the same HLA proteins on their surface is extremely small—about 1 in 10 million. These HLA antigens are a unique self-code expressed on every leukocyte in each individual's body. Although the exact function of the HLA-A, -B, and -C antigens is not completely understood, it is felt that the antigens from these three loci are critical in generating an immune response against virus-infected cells. The HLA-A, -B, and -C protein antigens may function in part as receptors for viruses. It is likely that the mononuclear phagocyte "sees" a virus in association with the HLA-A, -B, and -C antigens found on the infected cell as altered self. Presentation of these altered self molecules (viruses plus HLA-A, -B and -C proteins) to T lymphocytes activates a killer-T lymphocyte that will kill any virally infected cell. Because every body cell (except red blood cells) expresses HLA-A, -B, and -C antigens, any virally-infected cell should be recognized by the killer-T lymphocyte. Killer T lymphocytes are also generated in response to foreign HLA-A, -B, and -C antigens in HLA mismatched transplanted organs.

How can any given individual's self-code (HLA antigens) be determined? HLA-A, -B, and -C antigens are detected by reacting any individual's leukocytes with a panel of antibodies, each specific for one of the multiple HLA-A, -B, and -C proteins known. Each specific antibody will react with only one HLA antigen—the protein product of one allele from the HLA-A, -B, or -C gene. After determining the set of antibodies (Ig) with which a given individual's leukocytes react, a list of the HLA antigens on those leukocytes can be made. This laboratory procedure is called **HLA typing**.

At least three classes of proteins are coded for by the *class II* HLA genes; they are called **DP, DQ,** and **DR**. We will not review the DP and DQ genes or their protein products in this text because their exact function in humans is not currently known. The DR antigens are coded for by two genes that lie close to the HLA-A, -B, and -C gene regions on chromosome #6. One DR gene codes for a light protein chain; at least 14 alleles are known to exist for this light DR protein chain gene site. Next to the gene site for the **light DR protein chain** is a gene site for a **heavy DR protein chain**. No alleles at this gene site are currently known, thus only one type of heavy DR protein chain is known to be made. The heavy chain of DR is the same in all humans. The light protein chain of the DR is the only protein chain that has allelic variants. This chain, also known as the **polymorphic** (many shapes) **chain**, has at least 14 alleles (see Figure 22–2). The half of the light chain of DR closest to the cell membrane has an identical amino acid sequence in all humans; but at the terminal end of the light chain there is substantial variability in the amino acid sequences from one DR antigen to another (there are at least 14 known different sequences). Because both alleles at the two matching DR gene sites are coexpressed, two different DR protein antigens can be expressed on the surface of each leukocyte. Most cells in the body do *not* express DR antigens on their surfaces (in contrast to the HLA-A, -B, and -C antigens). Four cell types that are known to express DR antigens are the cells that make up the lining of the blood vesels, B lymphocytes, mononuclear phagocytes, and activated T lymphocytes activated T lymphocytes (but not unactivated T lymphocytes).

The principal cell for which the function of DR is understood is the *mononuclear phagocyte.* DR proteins have been found to play an important role in antigen processing and presentation. As shown in Figure 16–1, processed antigen must be presented on the surface of a mononuclear phagocyte in association with the DR proteins. In turn, T lymphocytes must have a receptor for the same DR protein that is found on the mononuclear phagocyte, in addition to a receptor for the specific antigen itself, in order for activation of the T-lymphocyte clone to occur. It is felt that the T-lymphocyte antigen receptor and DR receptor may be a single receptor that recognizes the *DR protein that is physically*

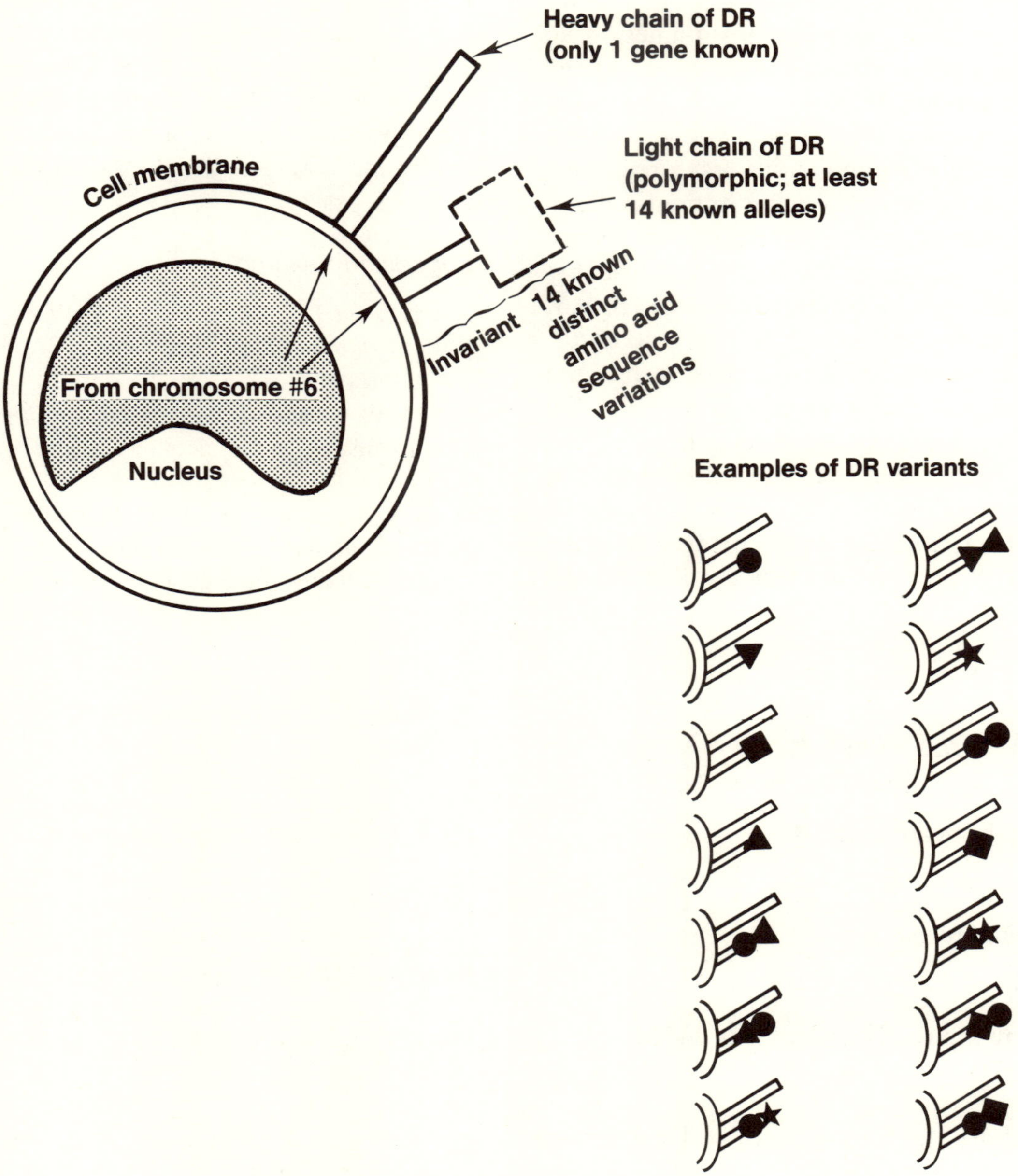

Figure 22–2. Details of DR antigen expression.

associated with processed antigen. A mismatch between the mononuclear phagocyte DR protein and the T-lymphocyte DR protein receptor (as might occur during *in vitro*, or *in test tube,* experimentation) will prevent the T-lymphocyte clone from being activated by processed antigen. The DR proteins expressed on any individual's mononuclear phagocytes (or B lymphocytes) can be deternined by the use of DR protein-specific antibodies, as discussed in the HLA-A, -B, and -C section.

The DR proteins are important for one other function besides antigen presentation. In laboratory experiments in which the leukocytes from two different individuls are placed in *culture* (removed from the body and maintained in an incubator), a distinctive reaction called a **mixed leukocyte reaction (MLR)** is observed. The mixed leukocyte reaction (MLR) occurs because two different leukocyte populations, each regarding the other as foreign, will begin to proliferate, a prelude to mounting immune responses against one another. Because the MLR response has been found to be totally unrelated to the HLA-A, -B, and -C antigens expressed by the leukocytes, it is now known to be due to a mismatch in the DR proteins (or the other class II proteins, DP or DQ) expressed by the two cell types. As shown in Figure 22–3, a mismatch between the DR proteins expressed on the leukocytes of one individual and the DR proteins expressed on the leukocytes of a second individual will create the *MLR* response: if two different individuals have the same class II proteins on their cell surfaces, no MLR response will occur. This test (co-culture of two individuals' leukocytes) is performed when possible prior to organ transplantation to determine how compatible the two individuals' cells are.

Suggested Reading

Hood, L. E., I. L. Weissman, W. B. Wood, and J. H. Wilson. *Immunology*. Menlo Park, CA: Benjamin/ Cummings, 1984.

Miller, W. V. and G. Rodey. *HLA Without Tears.* Chicago: American Society of Clinical Pathologists, 1981.

Stites, D. P., J. D. Stobo, H. H. Fudenberg, and J. V. Wells. *Basic and Clinical Immunology,* 4th ed. Los Altos, CA: Lange Medical Publications, 1982.

REVIEW QUESTIONS for Human Leukocyte Antigens (HLA)

1. What is meant by HLA?

HLA are Human Leukocyte Antigens. [p. 121]

2. How are the HLA antigens related to the immune response?

Individuals expressing certain HLA proteins on their cells tend to have certain types of specific immune responses. [p. 121]

3. Where are the HLA antigens coded?

HLA antigens are coded for on chromosome #6. [p. 121]

4. What are the three classes of HLA genes? What do they code for?

1) Class I HLA genes code for the HLA-A, -B, and -C proteins.
2) Class II HLA genes code for the HLA-DR, DP, and DQ proteins.
3) Class III HLA genes code for several proteins including the complement components.

[p. 122]

5. Approximately how many alleles are currently known to exist at the HLA-A, -B, -C, and -DR sites?

There are at least 23 alleles of HLA-A, 48 alleles of HLA-B, 8 alleles of HLA-C, and 14 alleles of HLA-DR. [p. 122]

6. What protein must be present with HLA-A, -B, and -C in order for those HLA antigens to be expressed on the cell surface?

Beta two (B_2) microglobulin must be present. [p. 122]

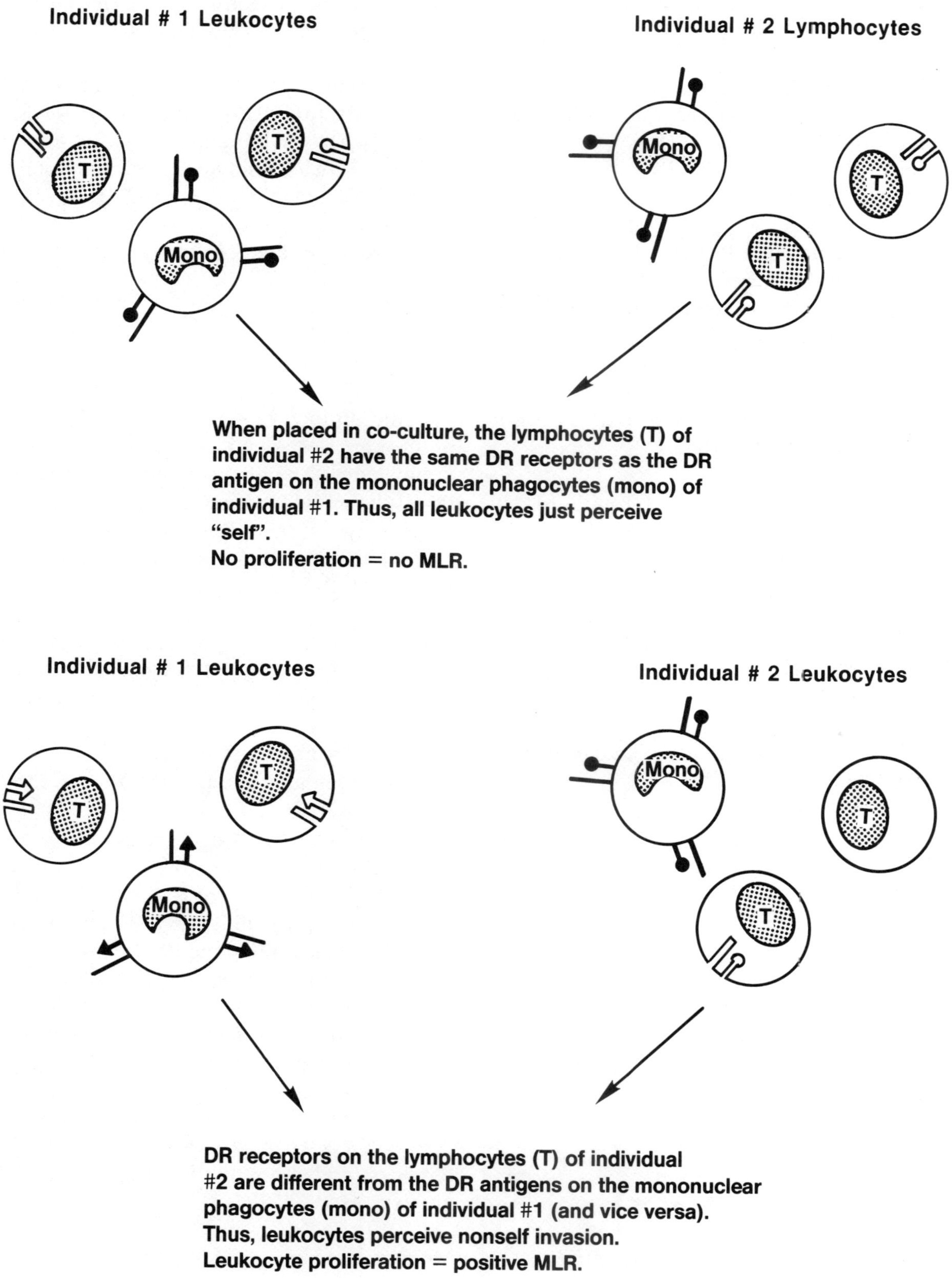

Figure 22–3. Mechanism for the mixed leukocyte response (MLR).

7. What cells express the HLA-A, -B, and -C antigens?

Most cells in the body express the HLA antigens, except the red blood cells. [p. 122]

8. What is the maximum number of HLA-A, -B, -C, or -DR antigens that an individual can express?

Each cell can express a maximum of two HLA-A, two HLA-B, two HLA-C, and two HLA-DR proteins. If the cell is homozygous for any HLA allele (has two identical alleles), only one type of that protein will be expressed. [p. 122]

9. If an individual inherits two different alleles at any given HLA gene site, how do those alleles interact (for example, recessive, dominant, or coexpressive)?

All HLA alleles are coexpressed. [p. 122]

10. How are HLA-A, -B, -C and -DR antigens detected on the cell surface?

Specific antibodies (Ig) for each HLA protein antigen are developed. An individual's cells are incubated with a panel of all the known antibodies. If the individual's cells react with any of the specific types of antibodies, it is then known that his or her leukocytes must express that specific HLA antigen. [p. 124]

11. What is th function of the HLA-A, -B, and -C antigens?

The HLA antigens are probably involved in generating immune responses against viruses and HLA mismatched organ transplants. [p. 124]

12. How many protein chains are found in the DR antigen?

Two protein chains (one heavy and one light chain) are found in the DR antigen. [p. 124]

13. What are some characteristics of the heavy chain of DR?

The gene that codes for the heavy chain of DR is on a chromosome next to the gene site for the light chain of DR. There is one gene known to be able to occupy this gene site. The sequence of amino acids is the same in all heavy chains of DR within the human species. [p. 124]

14. What are the characteristics of the light chain of DR?

The light chain of DR also comes from chromosome #6. However, at least 14 different possible alleles of DR are known to be able to occupy this gene site. The terminal portion of the DR light chain is where the various amino acid differences (coded for by the 14 different alleles) are expressed. [p. 124]

15. What cells express the HLA-DR antigen?

Mononuclear phagocytes, B lymphocytes, the cells that make up the lining of the blood vessels, and activated T lymphocytes express the HLA-DR antigen. [p. 124]

16. What is the function of DR proteins?

DR proteins found on mononuclear phagocytes play an important role in antigen processing and presentation. Specifically, DR proteins of the antigen-processing cell (the mononuclear phagocyte) must match the DR receptor on the responding T-lymphocyte clone. In addition, the T-lymphocyte antigen receptor must match the processed antigen on the surface of the mononuclear phagocyte. The T-lymphocyte receptor may in fact "see" only the DR protein in physical association with the processed antigen. [p. 124]

17. What is the MLR?

The MLR (Mixed Leukocyte Response) occurs when leukocytes from one individual are mixed with leukocytes from another individual of a different DR type. The leukocytes of one individual perceive the leukocytes of the other individual as nonself invaders and begin proliferating (a positive MLR). If the two individuals' leukocytes bear the same class II HLA antigens, no MLR will take place. [p. 126]

CHAPTER 23

USEFUL HUMAN IMMUNOLOGIC LABORATORY TESTS

In this chapter we will review certain tests that are performed on the serum and the leukocytes of patients to find out more about the function of their immune systems. These laboratory tests are designed to 1) characterize immunologic proteins found in a patient's serum, 2) classify the types of leukocytes found in a patient's bloodstream, or 3) better understand the function of these leukocytes. Due to their diseases, some patients display abnormalities in the types of immunologic proteins found in their serum or in the function of the leukocytes found in their bodies. However, these parameters usually return to normal following appropriate therapy.

Tests of Proteins (C and Ig) Found in Patients' Serum

There are several tests pertinent to the proteins found in patients' serum that are helpful in diagnosing and treating immunologic diseases. Because the *complement components* (C) are found in human serum, it is possible to measure directly the amount of each of the classical pathway complement components (C1 to C9) individually. In addition, tests have been developed to measure the ability of the complement cascade to assemble a functional membrane attack complex (as described in Chapter 19). One such test, known as the **CH50 test**, measures the ability of the complement components in a given patient's serum to **hemolyze** (poke holes in) red blood cells. Thus, it is possible to measure both the functional activity of the complement cascade and the concentrations of the individual complement components themselves.

The other main immunologic protein found in human serum is *immunolobulin (Ig)*. Recall that *protein electrophoresis* (reviewed in Chapter 5) provides an estimate of the total amount of gamma globulin (Ig) found in patients' serum. It is also possible to measure precisely the level of each of the five classes of immunoglobulin found in their serum. One commonly used technique of measuring serum immunoglobulin levels (**radial immunodiffusion**) is to react the patient's serum with a rabbit antibody (Ig) specific for the desired immunoglobulin class (IgG, IgM, IgA, IgD, or IgE). Under the proper conditions, when the Ig class-specific rabbit antibody reacts with the appropriate human immunoglobulin class, a **precipitation reaction** occurs. This precipitation reaction is seen as a cloudy material that can be measured by a variety of techniques to determine the amount of human immunoglobulin that reacted with the class-specific rabbit antibody. In addition to measuring immunoglobulin by *visual inspection* of precipitation reactions, the rabbit antibody can be tagged with a radioactive tracer and the amount of human immunoglobulin in a precipitation reaction can be measured by determining the amount of radioactive tracer found in the precipitate. These types of immunoglobulin determinations are known as **radioimmune assays (RIA)**. Alternatively, the rabbit antibody can be tagged with an enzyme. When the complex consisting of the human immunoglobulin–rabbit antibody–enzyme tag is incubated with the appropriate colorless enzyme substrate, a brightly colored product of the enzyme reaction occurs. The immunoglobulin levels are then measured directly from the amount of color produced in the reaction. These types of immunoglobulin measurements are known as *e*nzyme-*l*inked *i*mmuno*s*orbent *a*ssays (**ELISA**).

The three different testing methods for measuring immunoglobulin levels (visual preciptation reactions, radioimmune assays [RIA], and enzyme-linked immunosorbent assays [ELISA]) are summarized in Figure 23–1. As discussed in Part IV of this text, defects in the levels of complement or immunoglobulin may reflect specific immunologic diseases; the levels of these components usually return to normal following appropriate therapy.

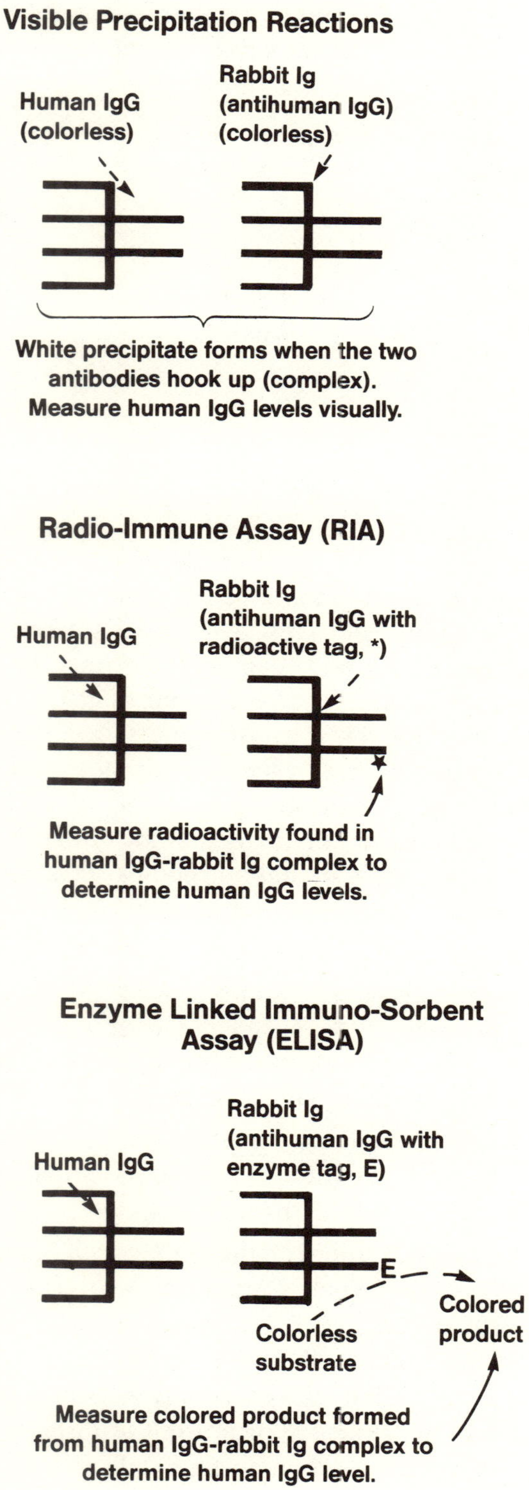

Figure 23–1. Three different methods for testing specific immunoglobulin levels (for example, IgG) in human serum.

Tests Designed to Classify Leukocytes

Monoclonal antibodies. A newly emerging methodology in the determination of leukocyte types in the blood involves the laboratory use of monoclonal antibodies (Chapter 14) to specific leukocyte membrane antigens. Monoclonal antibodies are made against various subsets of leukocytes. These antibodies include 1) **anti-monocyte** monoclonal antibodies; 2) **anti-B-lymphocyte** monoclonal antibodies; 3) **anti-T-lymphocyte** monoclonal antibodies; and 4) **anti-NK lymphocyte** monoclonal antibodies. There are currently two major competing commercial series of anti-human leukocyte monoclonal antibodies. One is the **Leu series** (Becton Dickinson Corporation) and the other is the **OK series** (Ortho Diagnostics Corporation). Both monoclonal antibody series have an **anti-pan T-lymphocyte monoclonal antibody** (that which recognizes *all* T lymphocytes) and **anti-subset T-lymphocyte reagents.** Although the numbering systems in the monoclonal antibody series are not analogous (as shown in Table 23–1), each company has monoclonal antibodies that react in similar fashions. The OK series is numbered as follows: **OKT3** recognizes an antigen found on all T lymphocytes, **OKT4** recognizes helper T lymphocytes, and **OKT8** recognizes suppressor T lymphocytes. In the Leu series, **Leu-4** is similar to OKT3 in that it reacts with all T lymphocytes, and **Leu-3a** recognizes helper T lymphocytes, as does **OKT4**. **Leu-2a** is the same as OKT8 in that it recognizes suppressor T lymphocytes. The comparison between the OK and

Table 23–1. Comparison of the Reactivity of Different Monoclonal Antibodies with T-Lymphocyte Subsets.

Monoclonal Antibody		
OK Series	***Leu Series***	***Diagnostic Application***
OKT3	**Leu-4**	**Identifies human T lymphocytes**
OKT4	**Leu-3a**	**Identifies helper T-lymphocyte subset**
OKT8	**Leu-2a**	**Identifies suppressor/killer T-lymphocyte subsets**

Leu series anti-T lymphocyte monoclonal antibodies is summarized in Table 23–1. Monoclonal antibodies also exist that identify B and NK lymphocytes and mononuclear phagocytes.

The ability of a leukocyte to bind a specific monoclonal antibody can be determined by various techniques. One very sophisticated instrument used for this purpose is a device known as the flow cytometer or **fluorescence activated cell sorter (FACS)**. This machine is able to separate cells that bear a specific membrane antigen (recognized by monoclonal antibodies) from other cells that do not bear that antigen. As shown in Figure 23–2, the FACS works as follows:

1) A mixture of cells, some bearing desired antigen, others not, is reacted with an antigen-specific monoclonal antibody that has been labeled with a **fluorescent tag.**
2) After a few minutes, the antigen-positive cells will bind the fluorescent monoclonal antibody; the rest of the cells will not.
3) The FACS then channels the cell mixture into a single-cell stream and analyzes each cell in turn for the amount of fluorescent monoclonal antibody that it bears.
4) The FACS analyzes not only whether a cell bears fluorescence or not but also the intensity of fluorescence on each cell.

Thus, the FACS analyzes a mixture of leukocyte cell types taken from human blood and determines the precise numbers of subset cells (T, B, NK cells, and monocytes). In addition, if needed, the FACS can separate (sort) the fluorescent cells (antigen-positive) from the nonfluorescent cells (antigen-negative) for further laboratory testing. The FACS is applied to the diagnosis and evaluation of immunologic diseases and treatment with increasing frequency. Alternatively, the cells that reacted with a fluorescent monoclonal antibody can be counted by the human eye by placing the cells under a **fluorescent microscope**.

Cell markers. In addition to the use of monoclonal antibodies batteries of other laboratory tests (based on distinctive functional characteristics of each leukocyte type—cell markers) can be performed to help confirm the type of any given leukocyte (Figure 23–3). One of these tests is the **SRBC-rosette assay**. An unknown type of mononuclear leukocyte is mixed with *s*heep *r*ed *b*lood *c*ells (SRBC). Because (for unclear reasons) T lymphocytes bear receptors for sheep red blood cells (SRBC), if a leukocyte binds with the SRBCs to form a *rosette* (essentially a cell covered with SRBCs), then it is probably a T lymphocyte bearing an SRBC receptor. A second test is the **assay for surface immunoglobulins (sIg)**. An anti-human sIg immunoglobulin is isolated from the serum of mice or rabbits, tagged with a fluorescent marker, and added to a mixture of leukocytes to see which cells become covered with this marker. The fluorescent anti-human sIg immunoglobulin binds only to those leukocytes that have sIg on their surface—*B lymphocytes*. B lymphocytes will glow with fluorescence under a fluorescent microscope, in

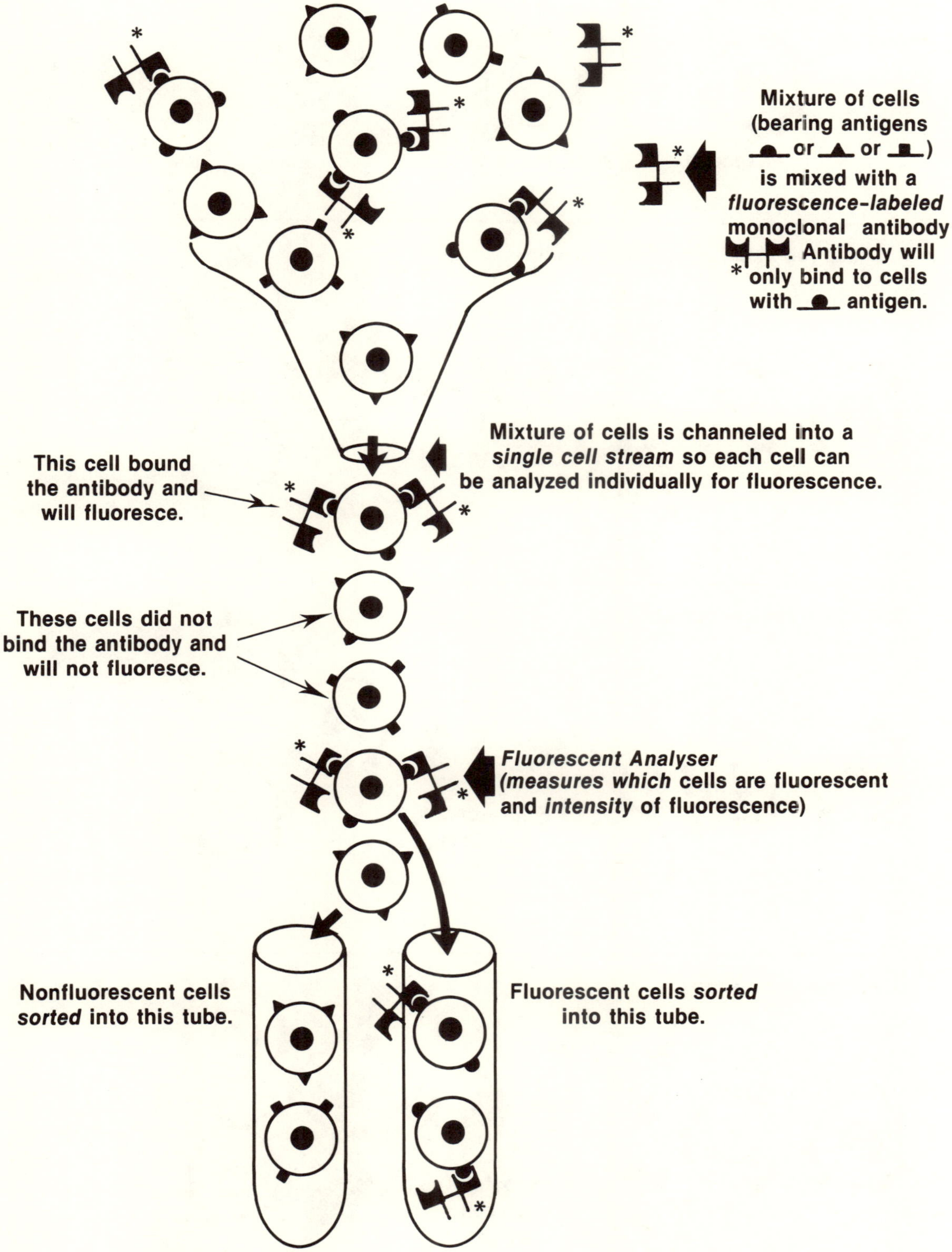

Figure 23–2. How leukocyte antigens are identified with a monoclonal antibody and the fluorescence-activated cell sorter (FACS).

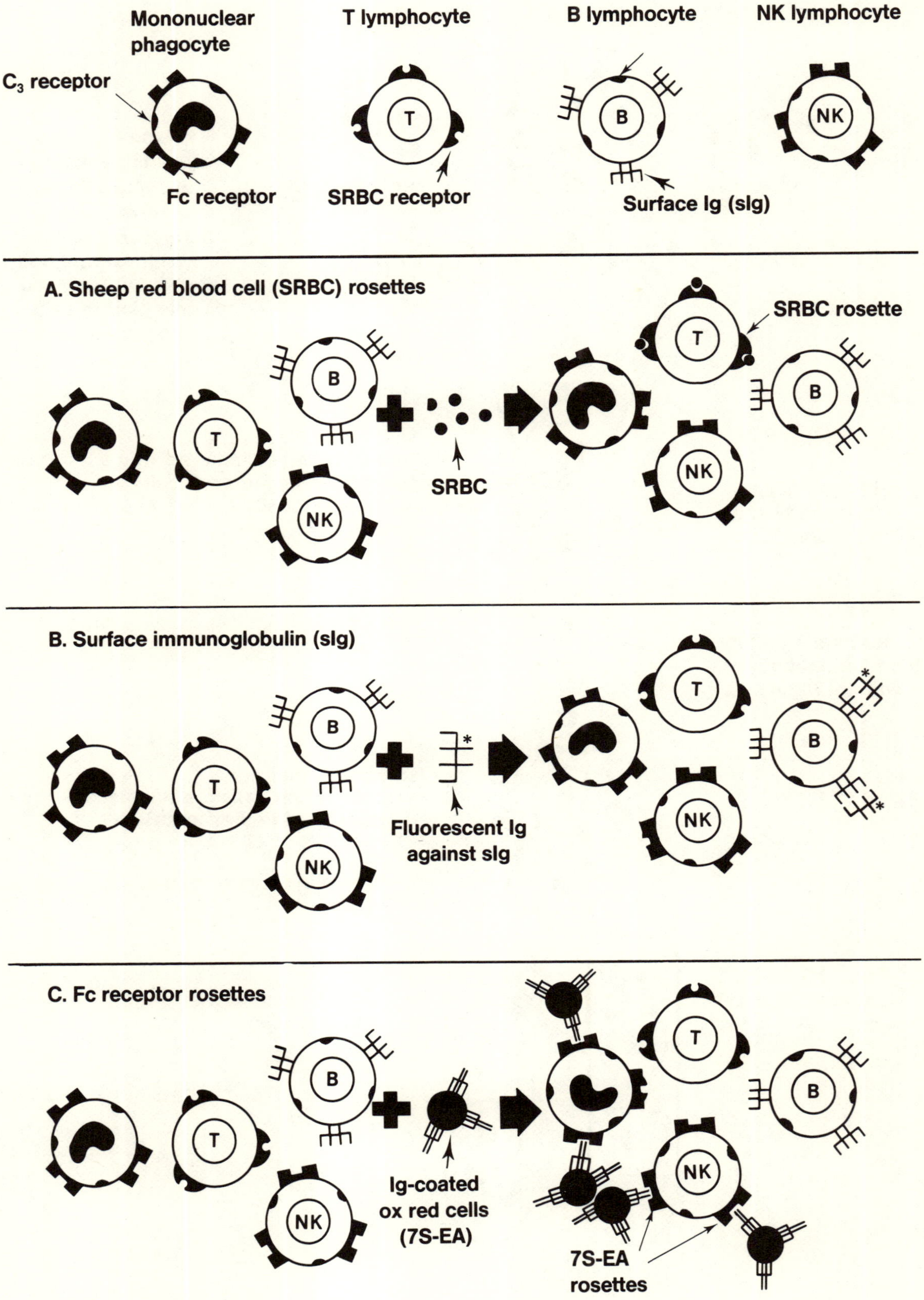

Figure 23–3. Six frequently performed identification tests for T, B, and NK lymphocytes and mononuclear phagocytes.

D. C_3 (complement) receptor

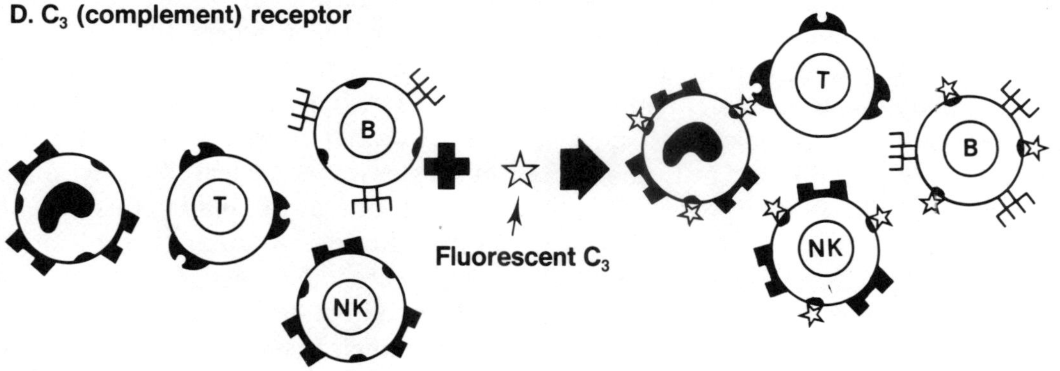

E. Phagocytosis

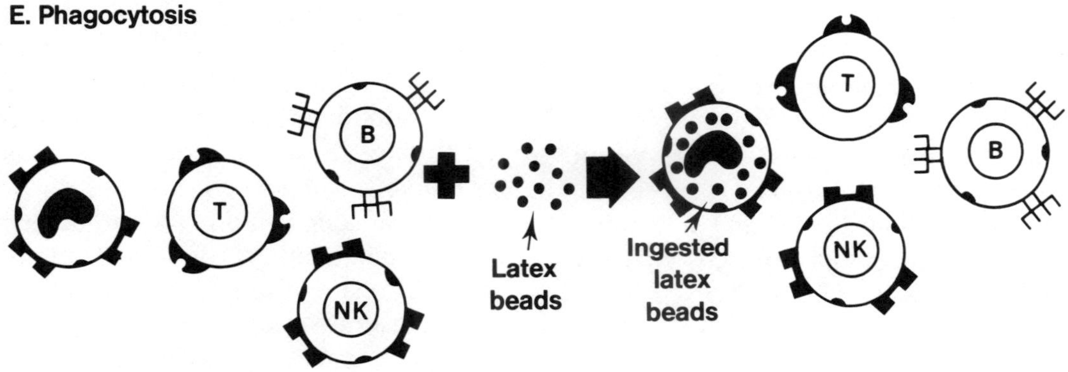

F. Esterase staining

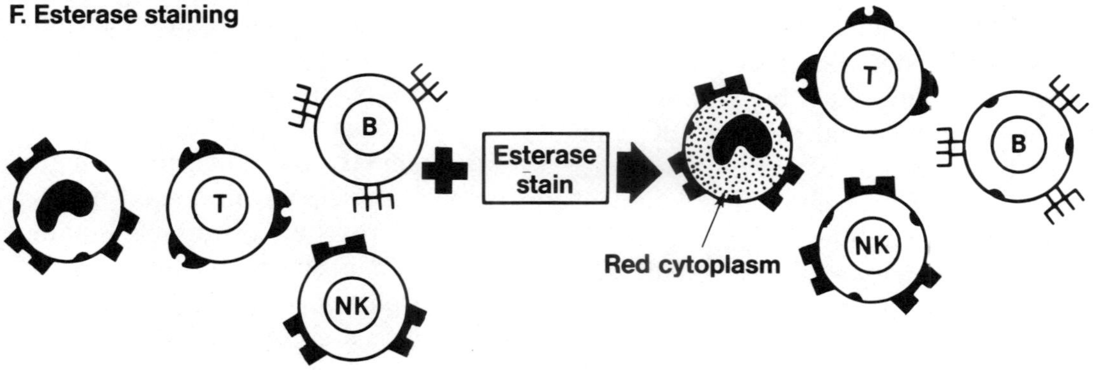

contrast to those cells that do not bind the anti-sIg immunoglobulin reagent. Any cells that have IgG nonspecifically stuck to Fc receptors on their membranes will also be identified by this technique. To remedy this problem, B lymphocytes and Fc receptor-bearing leukocytes (such as monocytes) are incubated in the test tube at body temperature for a few hours. After a few hours of culture, any Fc receptor bound antibody is shed from the membrane surface while the B lymphocytes continue active synthesis of new sIg.

Another test involves the **IgG Fc receptors** on the surface of certain leukocytes. Certain cells in a leukocyte preparation taken from human blood have Fc receptors on their cell membranes for the Fc portion of Ig. Of the four cell populations in a mixture of mononuclear leukocytes—mononuclear phagocytes, B lymphocytes, T lymphocytes, and NK lymphocytes—subsets of all four groups of cells possess IgG Fc receptors. However, just a *small* subset of B and T lymphocytes bear IgG Fc receptors, whereas virtually all monocytes and NK lymphocytes have IgG Fc receptors. Thus, possession of an IgG Fc receptor is not diagnostic of any one cell type but is still a valuable cell marker assay. Fc receptors on a leukocyte surface are identified in the following way: When rabbit antibodies (Ig) reactive with ox red blood cells (RBC) are mixed with ox RBC, an antigen-antibody complex is formed. When this rabbit antibody–ox RBC complex is incubated at 37°C with leukocytes possessing an IgG Fc receptor, interaction of the Fc portion of the antibody bound to the ox RBC with the Fc receptor on the cell membrane takes place and a *rosette* is formed.

A test to determine which leukocytes have *receptors for complement components* (specifically C3 proteins) focuses on isolating the C3 protein and the subsequent tagging of C3 to a fluorescent or radioactive marker. The tagged C3 is then mixed with leukocytes; those cells that have C3 receptors will bind to the tagged C3 and demonstrate radioactivity or fluorescence. Cells that possess C3 receptors include a large percentage of B lymphocytes, mononuclear phagocytes (probably the majority of monocytes possess C3 receptors), and some NK lymphocytes.

Tests for **phagocytosis**, the act of ingesting a target, are performed with two different types of targets. One type of target cell that can be used is an *Ig-coated ox red blood cell*. The phagocytic leukocytes (mononuclear phagocytes) possess an Fc receptor that will bind to this target and lead to its ingestion. Another type of target that is used is *latex (rubber-like) beads*. For some poorly understood reason, certain types of cells, such as mononuclear phagocytes, have receptors for latex beads and will **phagocytize** (**ingest**) the beads. However, mononuclear phagocytes cannot **digest** the beads. When the cells are viewed under a light microscope, their cytoplasm is seen to be filled with latex beads. The only population of mononuclear leukocytes that is felt to have these phagocytic functions are the *mononuclear phagocytes*.

Esterase stain is a test used to determine leukocyte classification. Mononuclear phagocytes (monocytes) contain a cytoplasmic enzyme called **esterase** that is capable of converting certain chemicals (α-naphyl butyrate and hexazotized parasinolin) into a red insoluble precipitate that can be recognized by inspection of the cells under a standard light microscope. Monocytes stain *red* when tested with esterase stain; other leukocyte subsets will not stain with the esterase stain.

In summary, the standard cell marker laboratory tests for classifying leukocyte types include: 1) SRBC-rosette; 2) surface immunoglobulin (sIg); 3) Fc receptors; 4) complement (C3) receptors; 5) phagocytosis; and 6) esterase staining. These tests are summarized in Table 23–2.

Laboratory Tests of Leukocyte Function

Cytotoxicity. Three cell types—mononuclear phagocytes, polymorphonuclear granulocytes (PMN), and NK lymphocytes—nonspecifically kill a wide range of target cells both spontaneously and by antibody-dependent cellular cytotoxicity (ADCC) (Chapter 20). Other cells—antigen-specific killer T-lymphocyte clones—kill only

Table 23–2. Comparison of Leukocyte Identification Test Results for B, T, and NK Lymphocytes and Mononuclear Phagocytes.

Cell	*SRBC-Rosette*	*Surface Immuno-globulin*	*Fc Receptor*	*C3 Receptor*	*Phagocytosis*	*Esterase Staining*
T lymphocyte	**Positive**	**Negative**	**Some positive**	**Negative**	**Negative**	**Negative**
B lymphocyte	**Negative**	**Positive**	**Some positive**	**Some positive**	**Negative**	**Negative**
Mononuclear phagocyte	**Negative**	**Negative**	**Positive**	**Positive**	**Positive**	**Positive**
NK lymphocyte	**Negative**	**Negative**	**Positive**	**Positive**	**Negative**	**Negative**

specific types of target cells (Chapter 17). The measurement of tumor cell killing *in vitro* (in the test tube) is called *cytotoxicity testing*. Patient leukocytes are tested in cytotoxicity assays to provide information about the immunologic function of the patient. Certain patients display defects in mononuclear phagocyte, PMN, NK, or T lymphocyte cytotoxicity. These defects are often improved following appropriate therapy (see Part IV).

Antigen-driven leukocyte functions. Chapters 16 through 19 reviewed the events following human immunization with a specific antigen. It is possible to duplicate these *in vivo* (in life) phenomena by placing a sample of a patient's leukocytes in test tubes with a specific antigen. Only a single clone of B or T lymphocytes will respond to each antigen used. Antigen-driven *B-lymphocyte* function can be monitored by measuring the amount of Ig that is secreted *in vitro* (in a test tube), by a variety of techniques. Antigen-driven T-and B-lymphocyte proliferation can also be measured. Certain patients demonstrate defects in antigen-driven B- and T-lymphocyte function, which can be corrected following appropriate therapy, as discussed in Part IV.

Mitogen-driven leukocyte functions. In the previous section, tests of antigen-specific B-and T-lymphocyte responses were outlined. Another type of immune system stimulator called the **mitogens** is frequently utilized in laboratory tests of the immune system. Mitogens are a class of compounds that activate most clones of B and T lymphocytes; they are **polyclonal activators**. There is very little immunologic specificity with mitogens. Some mitogens predominantly stimulate B-lymphocyte clones, while others predominantly activate T-lymphocyte clones. For the most part, addition of mitogens causes polyclonal lymphocyte activation. The best characterized mitogens are a class of compounds known as **lectins**. Lectins are proteins that have at least two identical subunits (divalent). These subunits have a pocket (receptor) that recognizes a specific sugar. The three lectins commonly used as mitogens in human immunology diagnostic research are **concanavalin A (Con A)**, **phytohemagglutinin (PHA)**, and **pokeweed mitogen (PWM)**. The receptor areas of these lectin proteins are lined with R groups, and the charges of the R groups have affinities for very specific sugars. For example, *PWM* recognizes a specific sugar known as N-acetylglucosamine, and any cell that bears an N-acetylglucosamine will be bound by PWM. As shown in Figure 23–4, after PWM binds to the sugar found on the leukocyte membrane, the entire antigen-processing system is bypassed and all lymphocyte clones are *directly*

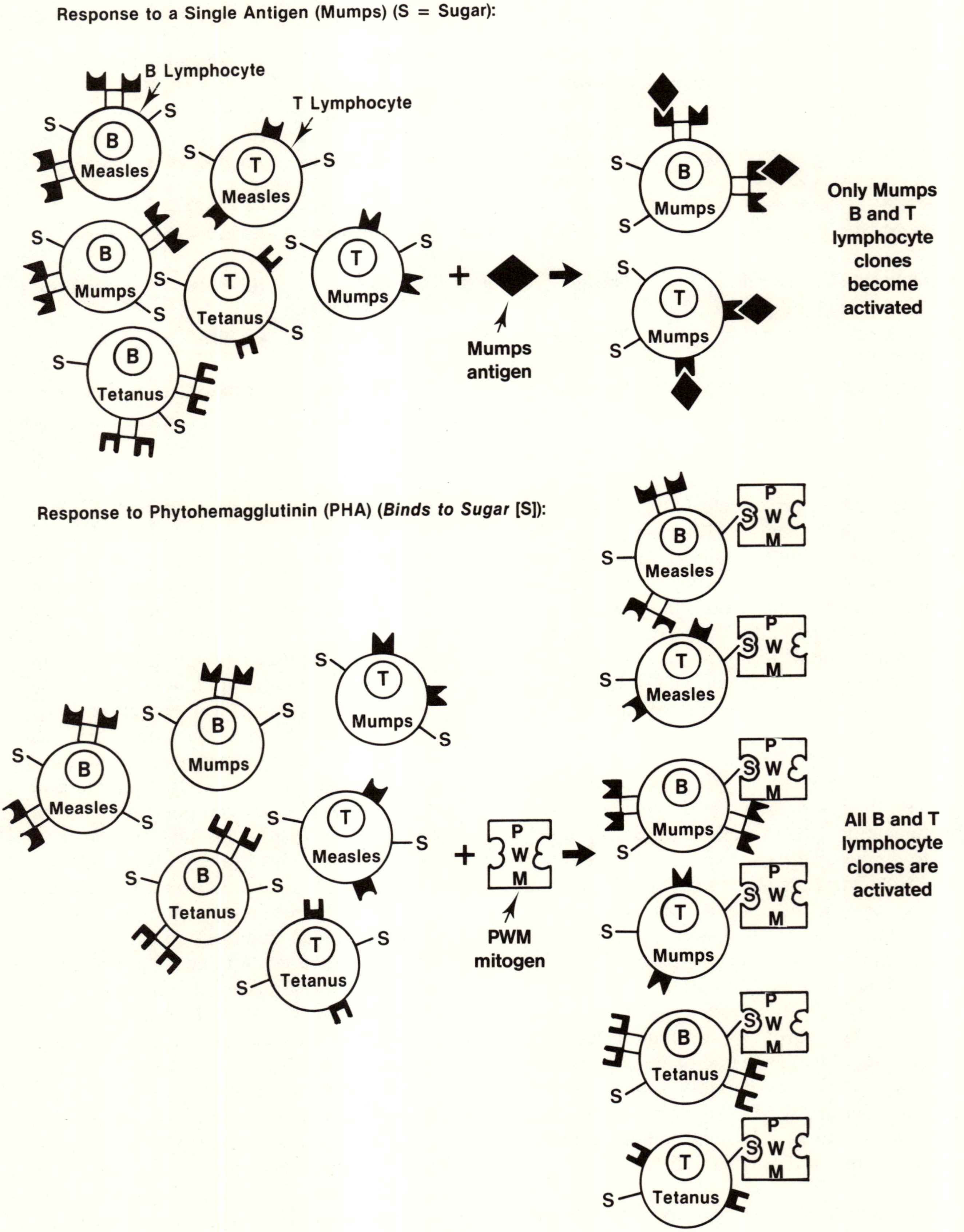

Figure 23–4. Differences between antigen- and mitogen-driven lymphocyte proliferation.

stimulated to proliferate. There is no clonal specificity to PWM-driven lymphocyte proliferation. Frequently measured mitogen-driven leukocyte functions include *B- and T-lymphocyte* proliferation and *B-lymphocyte* production of Ig in response to mitogen stimulation. Certain patients with immunologic diseases demonstrate characteristic defects in mitogen-driven leukocyte responses, which can be corrected following appropriate therapy.

Suggested Reading

Barrett, J. T. *Textbook of Immunology*. St. Louis, MO: Mosby, 1983.

Stites, D. P., J. D. Stobo, H.H. Fudenberg, and J. V. Wells. *Basic and Clinical Immunology*, 4th ed. Los Altos, CA: Lange Medical Publications, 1982.

REVIEW QUESTIONS for Useful Human Immunologic Laboratory Tests

1. What are the two main immunologic proteins found in human serum that can be measured?

   Complement (C) and immunoglobulin (Ig) can be measured. [p. 130]

2. What complement determinations can be made?

   Individual complement component (C1–C9) levels and total functional complement (CH50) can be determined. [p. 130]

3. What immunoglobulin determinations can be made?

   Levels of total Ig and each of the Ig classes (IgG, IgM, IgA, IgD, and IgE) can be determined. [p. 130]

4. What are two major competing series of monoclonal antibodies that recognize T-lymphocyte subsets?

   The Leu series and the OK series recognize T-lymphocyte subsets. [p. 131]

5. What monoclonal antibodies recognize all T lymphocytes?

   OKT3 and Leu-4 recognize all T lymphocytes. [p. 131]

6. What monoclonal antibodies recognize helper T lymphocytes?

   OKT4 and Leu-3a recognize helper T lymphocytes. [p. 131]

7. What monoclonal antibodies recognize suppressor T lymphocytes?

   OKT8 and Leu-2a recognize suppressor T lymphocytes. [p. 131]

8. What is a fluorescence-activated cell sorter?

   The fluorescence-activated cell sorter (FACS) is an instrument used to determine the number and fluorescence intensity of cells binding a specific monoclonal antibody. It also sorts out the cells that bind to the monoclonal antibody. [p. 132]

9. How does the FACS work?

A mixture of leukocytes is reacted with a fluorescence-tagged monoclonal antibody. Only leukocytes bearing a particular antigen will bind the monoclonal antibody. The FACS then channels the cell mixture into a single-cell stream and each cell is measured as to whether it fluoresces and (if so) with how much intensity. The FACS can sort the fluorescent (antigen-positive) cells from the nonfluorescent (antigen-negative) cells. [p. 132]

10. What are two additional identifying characteristics of a T lymphocyte?

A T lymphocyte is a lymphocyte that has SRBC receptors; subsets of T lymphocytes also have IgG Fc receptors. [p. 132]

11. What are some characteristics that identify a mononuclear phagocyte?

A mononuclear phagocyte is a phagocytic cell with a bilobed nucleus. It is esterase-stain positive and has IgG Fc and C3 receptors. There are also monoclonal antibodies specific for these cells. [p. 136]

12. What are some identifying characteristics of the B lymphocyte?

A B lymphocyte is a lymphocyte that expresses sIg. A few B lymphocytes express IgG Fc and C3 receptors. There are also monoclonal antibodies specific for these cells. [p. 136]

13. What are some characteristics of the NK lymphocytes?

NK lymphocytes are lymphocytes that do not bear sIg or SRBC receptors. They do have IgG Fc receptors. There are also monoclonal antibodies specific for these cells. [p. 136]

14. What are three forms of cytotoxicity?

1) ADCC (antibody-dependent cellular cytotoxicity)
2) Natural or spontaneous killing
3) Antigen-specific killing

[p. 136]

15. What cells can participate in ADCC?

Mononuclear phagocytes, PMN, and NK lymphocytes participate in ADCC. [p. 136]

16. What cells participate in spontaneous target cell killing?

Mononuclear phagocytes, PMN, and NK lymphocytes participate in spontaneous target cell killing. [p. 136]

17. What cells participate in antigen-specific target cell killing?

Antigen-specific killer T lymphocytes participate in antigen-specific target cell killing. [p. 136]

18. What is a mitogen?

A mitogen is a substance that will nonspecifically cause a large number of lymphocyte clones to proliferate. [p. 137]

19. Name three mitogens.

1) Phytohemagglutinin (PHA)
2) Concanavalin A (Con A)
3) Pokeweed mitogen (PWM)
[p. 137]

20. How do mitogens work?

Mitogens bind to specific sugars on the surface of leukocytes and directly activate lymphocytes (bypassing antigen processing). [p. 137]

21. How are mitogen-driven lymphocyte tests different from antigen-driven lymphocyte tests?

Antigens activate only one clone of lymphocytes; mitogens are polyclonal lymphocyte activators. [p. 139]

CHAPTER 24

IMMUNOREGULATION

The formal definition of a **biological response modifier (BRM)** is any soluble substance that is capable of altering or modulating the immune system in one of two basic ways: either with a stimulatory effect or a suppressive effect. BRM are usually polypeptides released by immune system leukocytes. BRM are types of hormones that allow cells at one location to communicate with other parts of the immune system. Some BRM were considered in previous chapters. Recall that there are two major groups of BRM: the *lymphokines*—soluble factors primarily released by *T lymphocytes,* and the *monokines*—soluble factors released by *mononuclear phagocytes.* The *lymphokines* include such BRM as *B-cell growth factor (BCGF), lymphotoxin (LT), interleukin 2 (IL2),* and *gamma interferon* (IFN_γ). In addition, *NK lymphocytes* have been reported to release IFN_α plus a factor that kills tumor cells directly called **natural killer cell factor (NKCF)**. The major BRM that *B lymphocytes* release is *immunoglobulin (Ig).* The *monokines* include such BRM as *interleukin 1 (IL1), alpha interferon* (IFN_α), *colony stimulating factor (CSF),* and *tumor necrosis factor (TNF).*

Lymphokines are powerful signals to the rest of the immune system. As reviewed in Chapter 17, when IFN_γ is released by T lymphocytes it stimulates many different activities including an anti-viral state in responding leukocytes (to prevent viral infection) and increased spontaneous killing by mononuclear phagocytes. *IL2* is a growth factor released by a small subset of activated T lymphocytes that induces the proliferation of other T lymphocytes. *BCGF* is a growth factor for B lymphocytes produced by helper T lymphocytes. These helper T lymphocytes also secrete an additional lymphokine that boosts immunoglobulin (Ig) secretion by B lymphocytes called **B-cell differentiation factor (BCDF)**. Suppressor T lymphocytes secrete a factor(s) that shuts off Ig secretion by plasma cells. **Lymphotoxin (LT)** is a protein, secreted by the killer T lymphocytes, that kills tumor cells directly. NK cells secrete a different protein responsible for much of their natural killing function known as **natural killer cell factor (NKCF)**.

Monokines (secreted by mononuclear phagocytes) have an equally broad range of signal activities. IFN_α is a type of interferon that protects cells against viral replication and also boosts the cytotoxic function of NK lymphocytes. *IL1* is required for T-lymphocyte activation (along with processed antigen and the DR protein). *CSF* is a growth factor released by mononuclear phagocytes, signaling the bone marrow stem cells to produce more leukocytes. *TNF* is a protein, secreted by mononuclear phagocytes, that kills tumor cells directly.

The mechanism by which the immune system regulates its own functions is called **immunoregulation**. Once the body has been penetrated by a nonself invader, the immune system must be activated to eliminate the antigen. The function of antigen-specific B- and T-lymphocyte clones must be geared up (**up-regulated**) during the early immune response to antigen. As the antigen finally gets eliminated from the body, the B- and T-lymphocyte immune function for that antigen must be geared down (**down-regulated**). BRM play an important role in immunoregulation. Figure 24–1 is an overview of the immune response to a nonself invader cell. It includes most of the cellular participants shown in the master schematic of the immune response (Figure 21–1). In this Figure 24–1, however, the dashed lines represent the biological

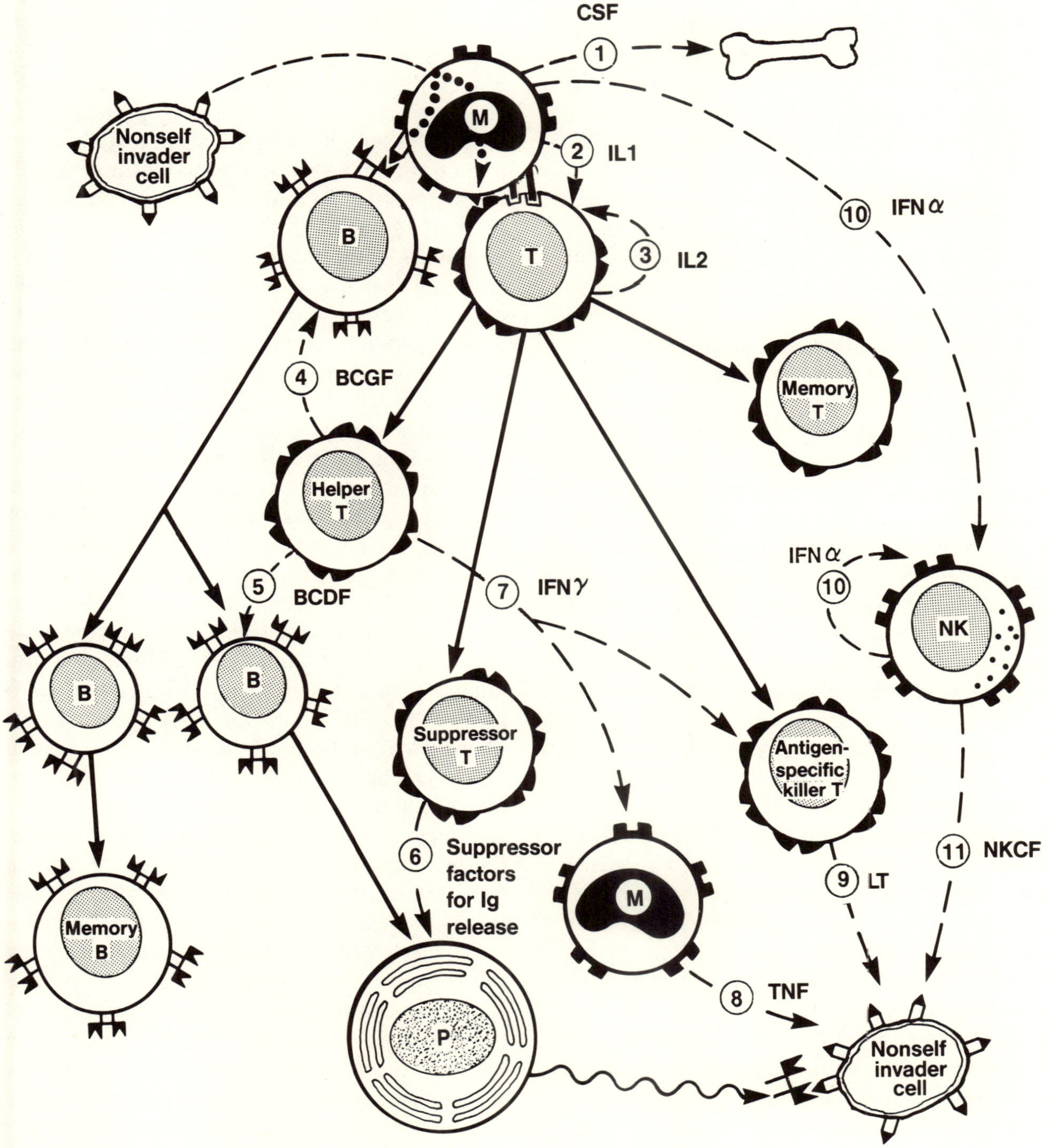

Key:						
	B	=	B lymphocyte	LT	=	Lymphotoxin
	BCDF	=	B-Cell Differentiation Factor	M	=	Mononuclear phagocyte
	BCGF	=	B-Cell Growth Factor	NK	=	NK lymphocyte
	CSF	=	Colony Stimulating Factor	NKCF	=	Natural Killer Cell Factor
	IFN_{γ}	=	Interferon (gamma)	P	=	Plasma Cell
	IFN_{α}	=	Interferon (alpha)	T	=	T lymphocyte
	IL	=	Interleukin	TNF	=	Tumor Necrosis Factor

Figure 24–1. Overview of immunoregulation.

response modifier (BRM) signals that are responsible for up-regulating and down-regulating the immune response. The 11 biological response modifiers that are reviewed in this schematic have been defined already. For simplicity's sake, an order in which the modifiers act and how they might cooperate in producing a concerted up-regulation of the immune response followed by appropriate down-regulation when necessary is indicated. Each specific biological response modifier is referred to by the number labeling it in the figure. Please refer to the specific area of the figure denoted by its number as you read the text.

The initiating factor for immune system activation is the interaction of the mononuclear phagocytes with the nonself invader cells. The antigens from the nonself invader cell become processed and are presented on the surface of the mononuclear phagocyte along with the two chains of DR. Some of the nonself invader cell antigens remain in their native (unprocessed) state on the mononuclear phagocyte surface. Once the mononuclear phagocyte becomes activated by the encounter with the nonself invader cell, one of the first monokines released is *colony stimulating factor* (#1—CSF). CSF travels to bone marrow stem cells to stimulate the production of additional mononuclear phagocytes. The mononuclear phagocyte releases *interleukin 1* (#2—IL1), a factor that cooperates with the processed antigen and DR to cause the activation of antigen-specific T lymphocytes. Once the T lymphocytes see the processed antigen in association with DR and receive the IL1 signal, they release a T-cell growth factor known as *interleukin 2* (#3—IL2). IL2 feeds back on the T-lymphocyte population to *expand their numbers* (by cell proliferation). One of the four T-lymphocyte subsets produced is the helper T lymphocyte (OKT4-positive) that releases a factor required for B-lymphocyte proliferation. This factor, known as *B-cell growth factor* (#4—BCGF), cooperates with the interaction of surface immunoglobulin with native antigen to induce the antigen-specific B-lymphocyte clone to proliferate. Once the B lymphocyte proliferates, it needs a second signal, termed *B-cell differentiation factor* (#5—BCDF). BCDF is a second helper T lymphocyte BRM that causes the proliferating B lymphocytes to become immunoglobulin-secreting plasma cells; memory B lymphocytes are also created. When immunoglobulin secretion is no longer required, the suppressor T lymphocytes (OKT8-positive) release *suppressor factors for immunoglobulin release* (#6—suppressor factors for immunoglobulin release). These suppressor factors interact at the level of the plasma cell to shut off immunoglobulin secretion. A third lymphokine secreted by the helper T lymphocytes is *gamma interferon* (#7—IFN_γ). IFN_γ promotes the differentiation of cytotoxic T lymphocytes. IFN_γ also stimulates mononuclear phagocytes to become markedly cytotoxic. Mononuclear phagocytes then release a factor known as *tumor necrosis factor* (#8—TNF) that directly kills tumor cells. In a similar fashion, the antigen-specific killer T lymphocyte (OKT8-positive) releases *lymphotoxin* (#9—LT), a lymphokine that directly kills tumor cells. Finally, natural killer lymphocytes are activated by *alpha interferon* (#10—IFN_α) both from mononuclear phagocytes and by auto-stimulation. The natural killer lymphocytes secrete a third protein capable of killing tumor cells, termed *natural killer cell factor* (#11—NKCF). Thus, immunoregulation refers to the overall interactions among the various participating leukocytes in the immune response. A great deal of the communication between these cells is accomplished by the secretion of biological response modifiers, both lymphokines and monokines. The overall functioning of the immune system depends on the *balance of helper and suppressor influences that are present at any one time*. Part IV of this text reviews *imbalances* of immunoregulation and their effect on immune system function.

Suggested Reading

Barrett, J. T. *Textbook of Immunology*. St. Louis, MO: Mosby, 1983.

Stites, D. P., J. D. Stobo, H. H. Fudenberg, and J. V. Wells. *Basic and Clinical Immunology*, 4th ed. Los Altos, CA: Lange Medical Publications, 1982.

REVIEW QUESTIONS for Immunoregulation

1. What is the definition of a biologic response modifier (BRM)?

BRM is a soluble substance capable of altering the immune response. A BRM can have either a stimulatory or suppressive effect on immune function. [p. 142]

2. What is a lymphokine?

Lymphokines are soluble factors (BRM) primarily produced by T lymphocytes. They direct other cells to perform specific functions. [p. 142]

3. What is a monokine?

Monokines are soluble factors (BRM) produced by mononuclear phagocytes. Monokines direct other cells to perform specific functions. [p. 142]

4. Give six examples of lymphokines produced by T lymphocytes. Describe their functions.

1) Interleukin 2 (IL2)—a growth factor for T-lymphocyte proliferation.
2) B-cell growth factor (BCGF)—released by helper T lymphocytes to cause B- lymphocyte proliferation.
3) B-cell differentiation factor (BCDF)—released by helper T lymphocytes to cause immunoglobulin secretion by B lymphocytes.
4) Suppressor factor(s) for immunoglobulin release (suppressor factor(s) for Ig release) —released by suppressor T lymphocytes to suppress immunoglobulin release by plasma cells.
5) Gamma interferon (IFN_{γ})—released by helper T lymphocytes to induce enhanced killing capabilities in mononuclear phagocytes. It also promotes killer T- lymphocytes differentiation.
6) Lymphotoxin (LT)—a protein capable of directly causing tumor cell death. It is released predominantly by the killer T lymphocytes. [p. 142]

5. Name four monokines and describe their functions.

1) Colony stimulating factor (CSF)—stimulates production of additional leukocytes by stem cells in the bone marrow.
2) Interleukin 1 (IL1)—a critical monokine that stimulates proliferation of T lympocytes.
3) Tumor necrosis factor (TNF)—a protein capable of directly killing tumor cells.

4) Alpha interferon (IFN_γ)—stimulates an antiviral state in tissue cells and causes enhanced killing capabilities in natural killer lymphocytes. [p. 142]

6. Name two lymphokines produced by natural killer lymphocytes, and describe their functions.

1) Alpha interferon (IFN_γ)—an antiviral agent that also is capable of activating natural killer lymphocytes to enhance tumoricidal activity.
2) Natural killer cell factor (NKCF)—a factor capable of directly killing tumor cells.

[p. 142]

7. Define immunoregulation.

Immunoregulation is the mechanism by which the immune system regulates its function. The function of the immune system at any given time reflects a balance of the helper and suppressor influences that are operating on the immune system leukocytes at that time. [p. 142]

8. Which are the principal cells responsible for up-regulating B-lymphocyte function? How do they work?

The OKT4-positive helper T lymphocytes secrete both B-cell growth factor (BCGF) and B-cell differentiation factor (BCDF). They work at different stages of the B-lymphocyte activation process. [p. 144]

9. Which are the principal cells responsible for down-regulating B-lymphocyte function? How do they work?

The OKT8-positive suppressor T lymphocytes secrete suppressor factor(s) of immunoglobulin release that act directly on the plasma cells to help shut down any further Ig release. [p. 144]

PART IV

DISEASES OF THE IMMUNE SYSTEM

The goal of the first three parts of this book was to present the basic concepts and terminology of immunology required for understanding the function of the human immune system. In Part IV the basic concepts are applied to those circumstances in which the human immune system does not function properly, specifically, the immunologic diseases.

In general terms, diseases of the immune system can be broadly classified from a functional perspective. The **allergic and hypersensitivity diseases** (Chapter 25) represent those situations in which the immune system appears to be overreactive to nonself molecules. The **autoimmune diseases** are clinical situations in which the immune system appears to be reactive against self molecules (Chapter 26). The **immunodeficiency diseases** (Chapter 27) represent those clinical situations in which there is a partial or complete defect in immune system function. In Chapter 28 we present some of the newer clinical forefronts of immunology, specifically **transplantation medicine** and **cancer immunotherapy**.

Three basic approaches to understanding immunologic diseases are presented in each clinical immunology chapter. First, we attempt to relate the immunologic defect of the disease to the basic immunologic physiology already presented in Part III. Second, we present certain of the chief symptoms and clinical findings associated with some of the representative diseases from each disease category. Finally, we outline some of the basic treatments that are used today. As with previous chapters, it is hoped that those readers with strong clinical interests will be motivated to refer to some of the excellent, more detailed suggested reading materials pertinent to each disease.

CHAPTER 25

THE ALLERGIC DISEASES AND OTHER IMMUNE HYPERSENSITIVITY STATES

The immune system functions by identifying self molecules as distinct from nonself molecules and destroying any nonself invaders. The immune system appears to be tolerant, however, to many nonself molecules that are only exposed to the surfaces of the body. These surfaces include the skin, the nose, the upper airways of the lung, the mouth, the gastrointestinal tract, and the mucous membranes covering the eyes (called the conjunctivae). Approximately 10 percent of individuals are intolerant of certain environmental antigens that touch the body surfaces. These individuals are *allergic* and they develop characteristic allergic immunologic reactions to certain environmental antigens known as **allergens**.

The two factors that characterize persons as allergic are: 1) they mount an immune response to environmental antigens (allergens) to which the remainder of the population does not react, and 2) the immune response that is produced is different from the immune response of a nonallergic or normal individual. Specifically, the B lymphocytes of allergic individuals secrete **immunoglobulin E (IgE)** that binds to the specific allergen. Also, allergic individuals ordinarily do not produce significant amounts of IgG or IgM antibodies to the allergen (the typical response of a normal person)—mostly IgE. The reason for this defect in immunoregulation is not known. As shown in Figure 25–1, once the allergic patient's B lymphocytes produce IgE immunoglobulins, these immunoglobulins circulate throughout the bloodstream until they come in contact with a type of cell called a **mast cell**.

Mast cells are found throughout the tissues of the body but are localized most heavily in the skin, the muscosal linings of the nose and the upper airways, the conjunctival lining of the eye, and the gastrointestinal tract. Mast cells are distinctive for two reasons: 1) they have numerous receptors on their cell membranes for the Fc portion of IgE (**IgE Fc receptors**), and 2) they contain numerous, potent inflammatory chemicals stored in their cytoplasmic granules and cell membranes. The three most potent inflammatory substances released by the mast cell are known as **histamine**, the **prostaglandins**, and the **leukotrienes**.

The stimulus for mast cell release of these substances (**mast cell degranulation**) occurs when a primed mast cell, which is a mast cell whose IgE Fc receptors are saturated with IgE molecules, comes in contact with the pertinent allergen molecule. When *two or more* of the mast-cell bound IgE molecules bind via their Fab regions to the allergen molecule, the mast cell degranulates—releasing histamine, leukotrienes, and prostaglandins. These three substances then act on surrounding blood vessels and other tissues and subsequently cause irritation, inflammation, and mucous production (in mucous membranes—such as found in the nose and lungs). The allergic reaction is recognized when the skin of an allergic individual is challenged with an allergen. Within a few minutes, the patient develops what is known as a **wheal and flare response**. The wheal consists of a raised, white area (*edema*—discussed in Chapter 10) at the site of allergen inoculation; the flare is a red halo of dilated blood vessels surrounding the wheal. The wheal and flare together are known as **hives**, or **urticaria**; each skin lesion is very itchy.

The **symptoms** which characterize each of the allergic diseases relate most closely to the **ana-**

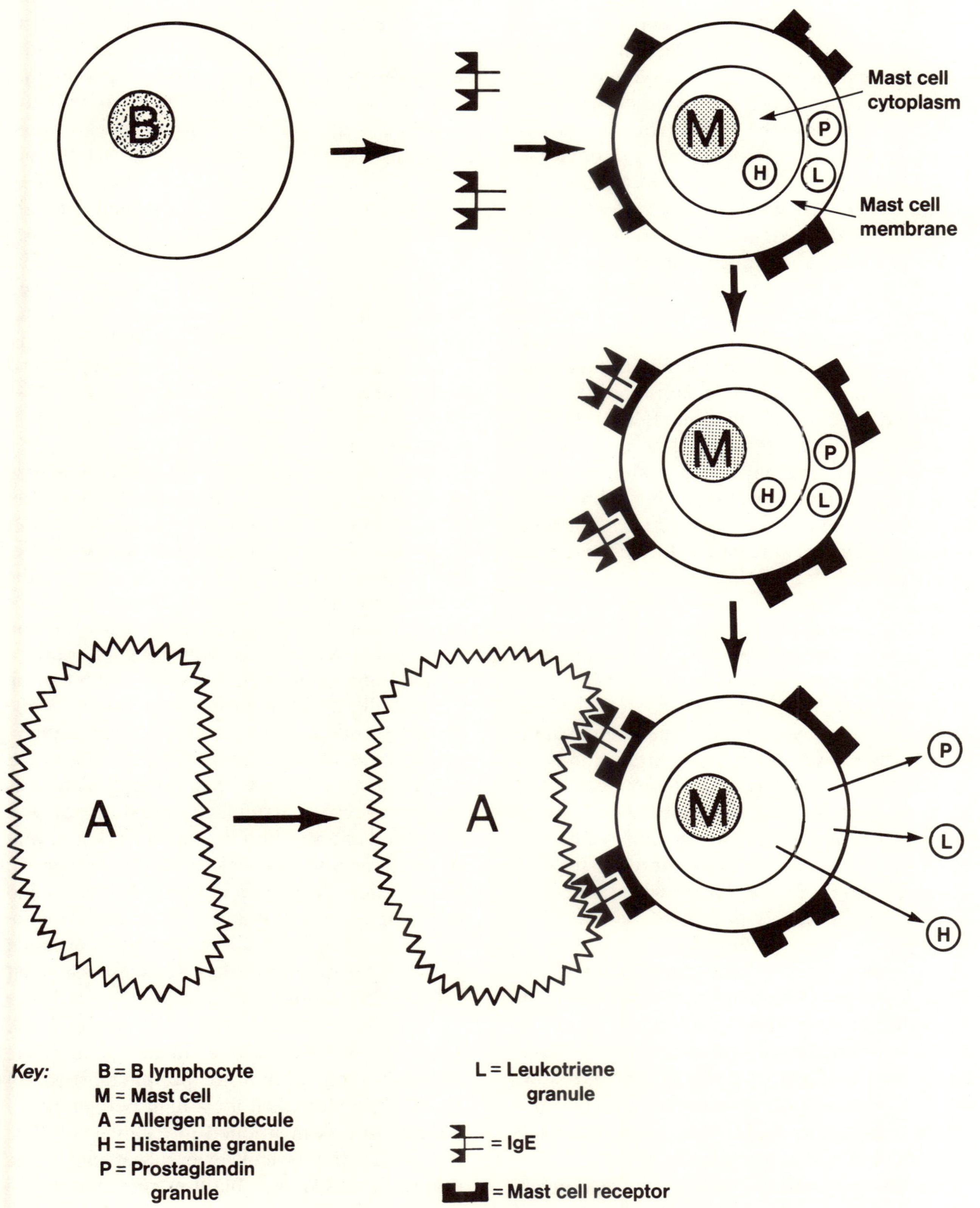

Figure 25–1. Mechanism for allergic reactions.

tomical site at which the allergens trigger mast cell release. The **actual mechanisms** of allergy are the same in each disease case. It is still not known why some patients have allergic symptoms confined to the nose as compared to others who have mainly symptoms in the lung and other sites. For example, when the offending allergen comes in contact with the eyes of certain allergic individuals, the conjunctival lining over the eyes becomes inflammed, reddened, itchy, and weepy. This condition is known as **allergic conjunctivitis**. When the allergen comes in contact with the nose, however, certain allergic patients may suffer from **allergic rhinitis (hay fever)**; this disease may present with sneezing, difficulty in breathing due to obstructed nasal passages, and an itchy nose with increased mucous production. If the allergen lodges in the lower airways of certain allergic individuals, **asthma** may occur. Asthma consists of increased mucous production in the bronchial airways coupled with the constriction of the muscles of the airway in response to the inflammation produced by histamine, prostaglandins and leukotrienes, from degranulated mast cells. This bronchoconstriction produces wheezing and shortness of breath. Moreover, bronchoconstriction can be so severe as not to allow adequate air exchange; this condition can lead to death if not rapidly reversed. Other allergic individuals may have allergies to certain foods. A **food allergy** occurs within minutes of ingestion of a certain food. Some of the symptoms consist of hives in the mouth or on the lips, diarrhea, bloating, and abdominal cramps. *Hives* or *urticaria* are the characteristic wheal and flare allergic responses, as described above. They occur when an allergic individual's skin is challenged with an allergen. Hives are localized where the allergen is rubbed into the skin, such as in skin testing that produces *local hives*. Hives are also a manifestation of an allergen distributed everywhere throughout the body, such as following the ingestion of an allergen, or after the intravenous injection of a drug to which the patient is allergic causing *systemic hives*.

The most serious allergic disease is **systemic anaphylaxis**. It occurs when an allergic individual ingests or is inoculated with an allergen to which he or she is very sensitive. Under these conditions, the allergen can travel everywhere throughout the body and cause mast cell degranulation everywhere in the body. It is not surprising that patients suffering from this condition will have systemic hives, asthma, gastrointestinal distress, runny nose, and itchy, irritated eyes. In addition, these patients can go into *shock*, a severe lowering of the blood pressure that can lead to death. Patients that exhibit symptoms of systemic allergic reactions are said to be in **anaphylaxis**. The serious nature of anaphylaxis cannot be overstated. It frequently occurs within a few minutes of allergen exposure, such as penicillin administration or an insect sting, and is frequently fatal without appropriate treatment. See Table 25–1 for a review of the symptoms of the various allergic diseases.

The diagnosis of allergic diseases can be very frustrating for both the patient and the physician. The history of the patient provides the most important diagnostic clues because many times the patient will not have any symptoms at the time of an office examination. A history of any of the symptoms cited in Table 25–1 that comes on rapidly and reproducibly following exposure to an environmental antigen should prompt suspicion of allergy. In many cases, purified allergy-testing substances are administered by a physician to detect the presence of primed mast cells in the skin of the patients. **Allergy skin tests** involve the superficial inoculation of the suspected allergen into the patient's skin, a wait of 15 minutes and a check to see if hives appear. If the patient develops a reproducible wheal and flare skin test reaction to any given purified substance, a suspicion of allergy can be entertained more seriously. Several **blood tests** also exist that might help establish a diagnosis of allergy. These include the measurement of the serum *IgE* level, which frequently is elevated in allergic individuals, and examination of the peripheral blood of the allergic individual for a high percentage of *eosinophils*, as mentioned in Chapter 12. The exact role of this leukocyte subset in allergic diseases is not known, but it is frequently found not only in the blood of allergic individuals but also in the nasal discharge of patients with hay

Table 25–1. Symptoms of Various Allergic Diseases of the Body.

Body Location	***Disease***	***Symptoms***
Eye	**Allergic conjunctivitis**	**Red, weepy, itchy eyes**
Skin	**Hives (urticaria)**	**Itchy, wheal and flare skin lesions**
Nose	**Allergic rhinitis (hay fever)**	**Itchy, congested, sneezy, drippy nose**
Gastrointestinal tract	**Food allergy**	**Mouth hives, diarrhea, bloating, abdominal cramping**
Lungs	**Asthma**	**Wheezing, short of breath, coughing (sputum production)**
Everywhere	**Systemic anaphylaxis**	**Can have all of above plus shock (leading to death)**

fever and in the sputum of patients with asthma.

The **treatment** of allergic diseases centers around three treatment modalities: 1) **avoidance**, 2) **desensitization therapy**, and 3) **drugs**. The treatment of choice, although frequently not possible, is *avoidance*. If, for example, a patient develops hay fever or asthma in response to a pet in the home, the recommendation is frequently made that the patient remove this animal from the home. Similarly, allergic symptoms that develop in the work place might require a change of job. Most importantly, individuals who develop allergic symptoms in response to drugs should be told to avoid those drugs at all costs. When avoidance is not possible, the patient may be treated with desensitization therapy, certain drugs, or both.

Desensitization therapy involves injecting the allergic individual with gradually increasing doses of the specific allergen to which he or she is allergic. This process of gradually increasing the immunizing dose takes many months to years. For reasons that are not quite understood, many allergic individuals treated in this fashion begin making an *IgG* antibody response to the allergen. This IgG antibody functions as a "blocking antibody" because it binds any allergen that the patient might come in contact with before that allergen can be bound by IgE molecules on the mast cell surface, thus blocking mast cell degranulation. Desensitization therapy can be uncomfortable, takes a great deal of time, and has the risk of inducing asthma or anaphylaxis if not properly performed. It is most effective in the treatment of patients with allergic rhinitis and bee sting allergy and is less effective in the treatment of the other allergic diseases. The drugs that are used to treat allergic symptoms will not cure the disease but will lessen the symptoms and make the patient more comfortable.

The most striking agents used to treat allergy are adrenalin and the adrenalin-like drugs. **Adrenalin** (**epinephrine**) is the first line of therapy for anaphylaxis and severe asthma and usually will produce dramatic responses within a few minutes. **Antihistamines** are chemicals (not antibodies) frequently employed in the treatment of allergic diseases. They work by competing for the histamine receptor sites on sensitive cells; thus, the histamine that is released by the mast cells cannot act on the blood vessels or other surrounding tissues. The last group of drugs that are employed in the treatment of allergy are known as **mast cell stabilizers**. The drugs in this category include the **corticosteroids** (such as **hydrocortisone**), the **theophyllines**, and **cromolyn sulfate**. Each of these drugs works by different mechanisms to prevent the mast cell from releasing its inflammation-promoting contents after it is triggered by allergen exposure.

In addition to allergic reactions, there are two other general types of *hypersensitivity* immune diseases to environmental antigens that can occur in the body: **immune complex diseases** (such as **serum sickness**) and **delayed hypersensitivity** diseases. Serum sickness occurs when an individual is injected with an antigen to which an IgG or IgM (complement-activating Ig) immunoglobulin response occurs. If the IgG or IgM binds to the foreign antigen *in the bloodstream*, a soluble *immune complex*—antigen plus bound immunoglobulin—is formed. As shown in Figure 25–2, these immune complexes float in the bloodstream until they are trapped in the capillary beds of the skin, the kidneys, the joints, and other areas. The most frequent symptoms of serum sickness are fever, skin rashes, painful joints, headache, and abdominal pain 6–12 hours after the intravenous infusion of an antigen, such as a drug. The inflammatory symptoms of serum sickness occur when the immune complexes become trapped in the various capillary beds of the body and *complement is activated* locally which destroys normal tissues. Once serum sickness develops, there is no effective therapy except to insure that the patient avoids future contact with the substance that produced it. Other immune complex diseases and their treatments are discussed in Chapter 26.

The final type of hypersensitivity reaction is called *delayed hypersensitivity*. Delayed hypersensitivity occurs when an individual reacts immunologically to environmental antigens by producing a *cell-mediated response* to that antigen, as shown in Figure 25–3. Such reactions are easiest to observe when they take place in the skin. Typically, a patient will complain of developing a skin rash 36–72 hours after exposure of

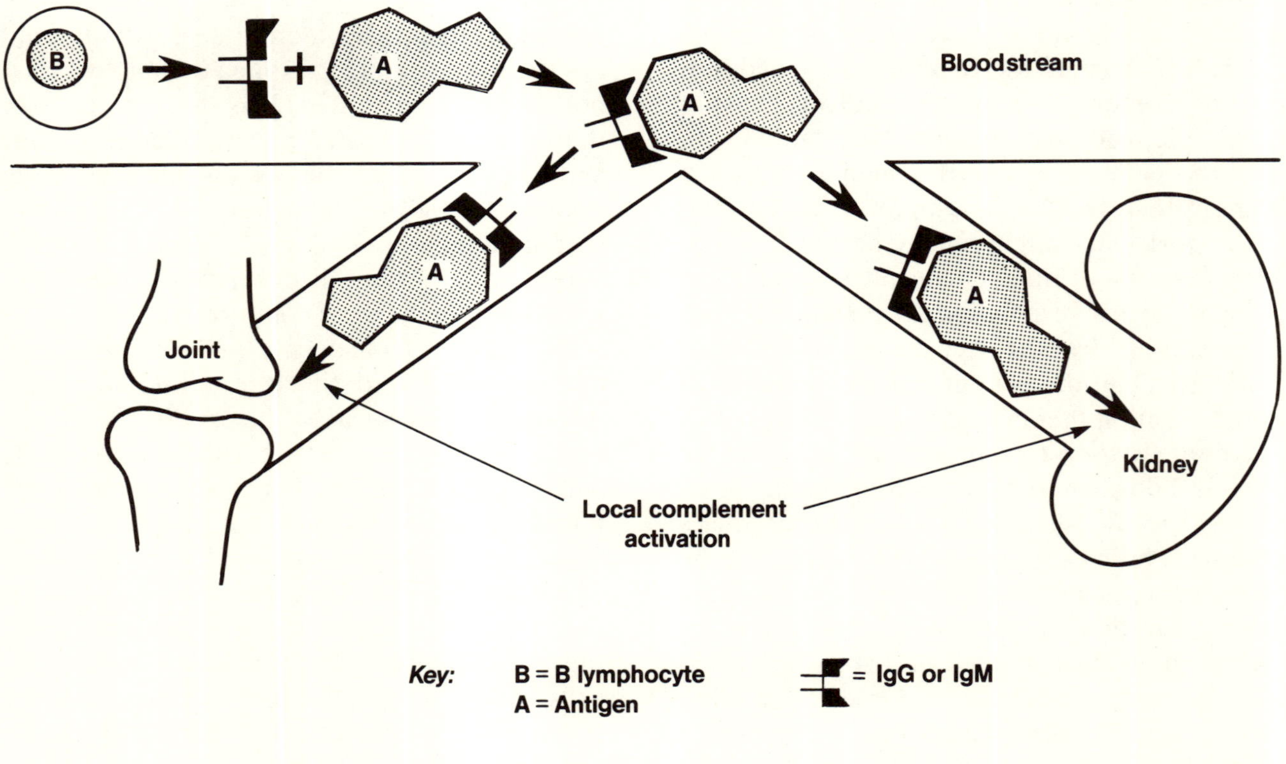

Figure 25–2. Mechanism for serum sickness.

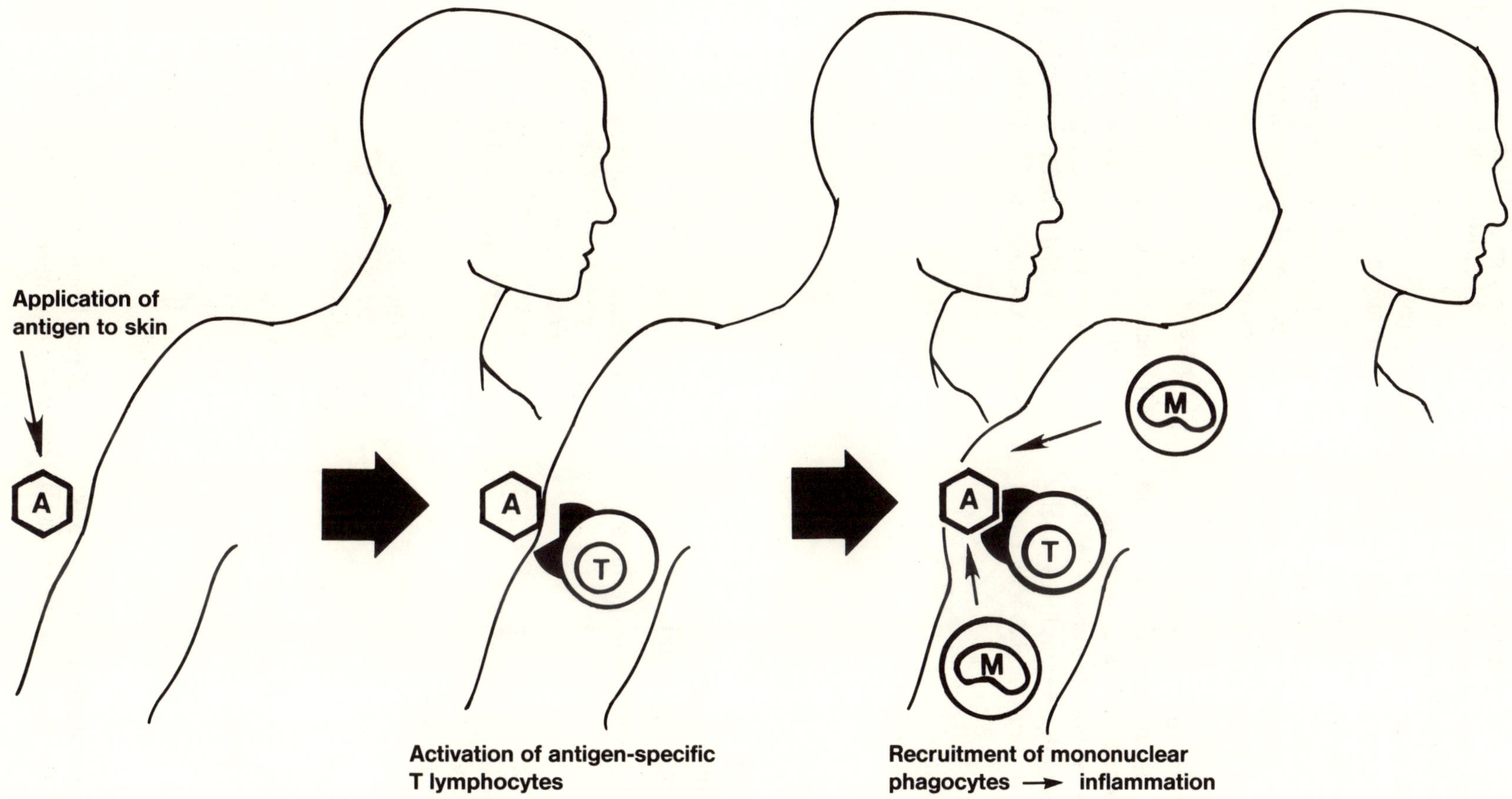

Key: A = Antigen
T = Antigen-specific T lymphocyte
M = Mononuclear phagocyte

Figure 25–3. Mechanism for delayed hypersensitivity skin reactions.

the skin to a certain substance. This rash is diffusely red, raised, and very itchy. Pathologic analysis of these lesions reveals antigen-specific *T-lymphocytes* and *mononuclear phagocytes* that have been recruited to the area of antigen exposure (as reviewed in Chapter 17). A typical example of delayed hypersensitivity skin reactions are those seen in patients reacting to *poison ivy*, certain types of *metal jewelry*, or certain soaps. The skin rashes from delayed hypersensitivity can be distinguished from the hives of allergic (IgE-mediated) reactions in three ways: 1) these rashes tend to appear as diffuse, red areas of skin rather than discrete wheal and flare reactions; 2) delayed hypersensitivity reactions take at least 36 hours to become maximal, whereas hives usually develop within a few minutes; and 3) a biopsy of delayed hypersensitivity reactions reveals that T lymphocytes and mononuclear phagocytes are present. In contrast, a biopsy of hives reveals primarily degranulated mast cells and local tissue destruction by mast cell-derived histamine, prostaglandins, and leukotrienes. Delayed hypersensitivity reactions may be treated by *corticosteroids* (see review of cortisone in Chapter 6). Avoidance of the offending antigen is usually recommended.

Suggested Reading

Middleton, E., C. Reed, and E. Ellis. *Allergy: Principles and Practice*. St. Louis, MO: Mosby, 1978.

Stites, D. P., J. D. Stobo, H. H. Fudenberg, and J. V. Wells. *Basic and Clinical Immunology*, 4th ed. Los Altos, CA: Lange Medical Publications, 1982.

REVIEW QUESTIONS for The Allergic Diseases and Other Immune Hypersensitivity States

1. To which nonself molecules is the immune system tolerant?

It is generally tolerant to nonself molecules that are only exposed to the surfaces of the body (skin, nose, upper airways of the lung, mouth, gastrointestinal tract, and mucous membranes covering the eyes). [p. 148]

2. Define an allergic individual.

An allergic individual does not tolerate certain environmental antigens that other people normally do, but instead develops characteristic immunological reactions to them. [p. 148]

3. Describe two factors that distinguish allergic individuals from nonallergic or normal.

1) They mount an immune response to allergens that other people typically do not.
2) The B lymphocytes of these individuals secrete IgE that will bind the allergens.

[p. 148]

4. Where does the IgE immunoglobulin go after it is released into the bloodstream by the B lymphocyte?

IgE gets bound to IgE Fc receptors found on the surface of mast cells. [p. 148]

5. Where are mast cells found in the body?

The mast cells are localized in the skin, mucosal linings of the nose and upper airways, conjunctival lining of the eye, and the gastrointestinal tract. [p. 148]

6. What are two distinctive features of mast cells?

1) They have receptors for the Fc portion of IgE.
2) They contain inflammatory chemicals stored in cytoplasmic granules and their cell membranes.

[p. 148]

7. What are three inflammatory substances released by mast cells?

1) Histamine
2) Prostaglandins
3) Leukotrienes

[p. 148]

8. What is the stimulus for the mast cell to release these inflammatory substances?

Two or more mast-cell bound IgE molecules bind to one allergen molecule. The mast cell then degranulates—releasing histamine, prostaglandins, and leukotrienes. [p. 148]

9. What is a wheal and flare response?

A few minutes after the skin of an allergic individual is challenged with an allergen, there develops a raised, white area (wheal) and a red halo around it (flare). [p. 148]

10. What are hives?

The wheal and flare skin reactions are known as hives or urticaria. [p. 148]

11. What do the allergic diseases all have in common?

Although the symptoms for the various allergic disease differ, depending on the anatomic site affected, the mechanisms of allergy are the same. In all cases, when the allergen comes in contact with the body, it triggers mast cell release of histamine, leukotrienes, and prostaglandins. [p. 150]

12. What are two other types of hypersensitivity immune reactions in addition to allergy?

1) Immune complex diseases (such as serum sickness)
2) Delayed hypersensitivity

[p. 152]

13. What is serum sickness?

This is a condition in which IgG or IgM is made in response to an antigen and binds to that antigen in the bloodstream. This immune complex (antigen plus antibody) ultimately becomes trapped in the capillary beds of the skin, kidney, and joints. Resultant symptoms include fever, rashes, painful joints, headache, and abdominal pain. [p. 152]

14. What is delayed hypersensitivity?

Delayed hypersensitivity occurs when an individual produces a cell-mediated response (T lymphocytes plus recruited mononuclear phagocytes) to an environmental antigen. When delayed hypersensitivity occurs in the skin, at least 36 hours following antigen exposure is required for a maximal skin rash to develop. [p. 152]

CHAPTER 26

THE AUTOIMMUNE DISEASES

When the immune system is functioning properly, it is able to distinguish nonself from self, and to eliminate any nonself invaders. The common thread linking all of the **autoimmune diseases** is that for some reason, immunologic mechanisms are activated which react against *self molecules*. With few exceptions, the mechanism for this aberrant behavior of the immune system is not known. Typically in the autoimmune diseases, a B-lymphocyte clone becomes activated to secrete an immunoglobulin bearing a specific idiotype region that reacts with certain self molecules. When an *anti-self IgG or IgM immunoglobulin (ASI)* binds to the specific self molecule, *complement*-mediated tissue damage may occur. In addition, *mononuclear phagocytes* may be recruited into the area. There is evidence that activated *T-lymphocyte* clones may play a role in certain autoimmune diseases. There is a wide spectrum of diseases that are typically classified as autoimmune diseases. The symptoms of the autoimmune diseases usually relate to the organ systems that are affected by the autoimmune process. Some examples of the autoimmune diseases and their treatment follow.

Perhaps the easiest of the autoimmune diseases to understand is *rheumatic fever*. Rheumatic fever can develop 7–14 days after an individual has been infected with **beta hemolytic streptococci**, a very *specific* type of bacterium. This infection usually takes place in the throat ("strep throat"). As the immune system attempts to respond to the beta hemolytic streptococci antigen, the appropriate *B-lymphocyte* clones make an IgM immunoglobulin with an idiotype region that will bind to this organism. This immunoglobulin response will be very effective as a mechanism for clearing the beta hemolytic streptococci from the body. Unfortunately, the immunoglobulin that reacts with the beta hemolytic streptococci also *cross-reacts* with an antigen that is found on *heart* muscle cells. Thus, as humoral immunity (IgM plus complement) combats the beta hemolytic streptococci, heart muscle cells are also damaged as innocent bystanders. The patient then suffers symptoms of heart inflammation and frequently develops irreversible heart damage. *Rheumatic fever is preventable* by eliminating beta hemolytic streptococcal infections with the appropriate antibiotics before the immune response gets a chance to make significant amounts of the ASI that cross-reacts with heart muscle.

In most other autoimmune diseases, the exact initiating cause for the creation of antiself immunoglobulins is not known. In the case of **autoimmune thyroiditis**, for example, the patient suffers from symptoms of **hypothroidism** (dry skin, edema, constipation, and feeling cold). These patients have B-cell clones that secrete antithyroid ASI which destroy *thyroid gland* function. Alternatively, in another thyroid disease (**Grave's Disease**), the patient suffers with an enlarged, tender *thyroid gland* and other symptoms of *hyperthyroidism* including agitation, weight loss, diarrhea, and other metabolic disturbances due to an overabundance of thyroid hormone. The cause of this abnormality is a *B-lymphocyte* clone that produces a specific ASI which binds with a particular receptor on the surface of thyroid cells. The antithyroid ASI reacts with thyroid cell membrane receptors and is called a long-acting thyroid stimulator (**LATS**). The thyroid cell is stimulated by LATS to release thyroid hormone, which causes many of the symptoms of the disease. Treatment of *autoimmune thyroiditis* principally consists of thyroid hormone replacement. Treatment of

Grave's Disease usually consists of trying to block thyroid function with certain drugs or by eliminating a large portion of the thyroid cells with surgery or radiation therapy.

Goodpasture's syndrome is a disease in which patients develop rapidly progressive *kidney* and *lung* failure, frequently fatal. For unknown reasons, these patients activate a *B-lymphocyte* clone that produces an ASI reactive against lung and kidney cells. These organs are frequently damaged by this immunologic reaction. Because this disease is so serious, *Goodpasture's syndrome* patients are frequently treated by the removal of large amounts of their **plasma** (serum that has been anticoagulated). Plasma is removed by a process called **plasmapheresis** in which as much circulating immunoglobulin as possible is eliminated from the blood. Poisonous toxins (such as **cyclophosphamide**) designed to kill most proliferating cells, particularly the proliferating B-lymphocyte clone that is producing the ASI, are also frequently administered.

Myasthenia gravis is a disease characterized by a progressive weakness of the *skeletal muscles* of the body. In this disease chemical signals released from nerves do not interact with specific receptors on the skeletal muscles required for normal muscle contractions. This disease can be very incapacitating and can be fatal if it affects the respiratory (breathing) muscles of the body. *Myasthenia gravis* patients have a defect in their immune system that allows a B-lymphocyte clone to produce an ASI that reacts with the nerve signal receptors at the junction between the nerves and the muscles—the **neuromuscular junction**. When these immunoglobulins bind to the neuromuscular junction receptors, they prevent nerve impulses from passing; thus the muscles cannot contract. This disease is treated with various drugs that attempt to boost neuromuscular junction function (such as **neostigmine**). Attempts are also made to decrease the ASI level in the blood by techniques such as plasmapheresis.

Some people are known to make immunoglobulins against the various *cellular components of the blood*. For example, if a person makes an ASI against **platelets (thrombocytes)**, **autoimmune thrombocytopenia** will result. These patients suffer from very low platelet counts, and bleeding can ensue. Other people make ASI against their own *red blood cells*, a disorder known as **autoimmune hemolytic anemia**. These patients suffer from low red blood cell counts and frequently require transfusions in order to survive. Also, certain people make ASI against their own *white blood cells* (leukocytes), a condition known as **autoimmune leukopenia**. These patients suffer from recurrent infections because there are not enough leukocytes available to fight off invading microorganisms. Finally, some people also make ASI against the *stem cells in their bone marrow* (from which red cells, platelets, and leukocytes are derived). These patients develop a condition called **aplastic anemia**, which means that they have decreased numbers of circulating platelets, red blood cells, and leukocytes. The treatment of the previously mentioned disorders centers around the removal of the offending ASI by plasmapheresis or by administration of drugs (such as cyclophosphamide) that inhibit ASI secretion by the B-lymphocyte clone. In some of these disorders **splenectomy** (surgical removal of the spleen) may be a helpful treatment because the spleen is a major site of immunoglobulin production and also contains numerous macrophages. Because of their IgG Fc receptors and phagocytic capabilities, macrophages are the dominant mechanism for clearance of antibody-coated targets.

There are several diseases in which **autoantibodies** are made, but they are not felt to be solely responsible for the symptoms of the disease. These diseases are considered *analogous to serum sickness* because they are *immune complex diseases*. The difference between these diseases and serum sickness is that no outside antigen is injected into the patients. Instead, the patients produce immunoglobulins against their *own tissue antigens*. In the disease called **systemic lupus erythematosus (SLE)**, patients produce immunoglobulins that react to their cell nuclei (antinuclear antibodies). These antinuclear antibodies probably do not account for much cellular destruction by themselves because it is difficult for the antinuclear antibodies to come into direct contact with the nuclei of living cells. However, in the normal wear and tear of the body, cells die and it is at this time that antinuclear antibodies form *immune complexes* with the nuclear antigens. This occurs in the patient's bloodstream. The antigen–antibody complexes then float to various capillary beds of the body and trigger local *complement* activation. The same tissue-destructive mechanisms are activated as found in serum sickness; normal tissue destruction occurs by the innocent bystander mechanism (see Figure 25–2). The tissues most frequently affected in SLE are the kidneys, skin, joints, and central nervous system. Treatment of this disease centers around drugs designed to disrupt B-lymphocyte secretion of ASI (such as cyclophosphamide); plasmapheresis is also used to decrease ASI levels in the bloodstream. Corticosteroids are also employed as a treatment of SLE.

Rheumatoid arthritis is a disease in which most patients produce an **IgM ASI** (rheumatoid factor) that reacts against *normal IgG* proteins circulating in the serum. The immune complexes formed, that is, *ASI plus normal IgG*, tend to lodge in the *joints* of the body, creating *complement*-mediated inflammation and joint destruction. Other tissues that can be affected in rheumatoid arthritis include the skin and the blood vessels. Treatment of rheumatoid arthritis centers around the use of various anti-inflammatory drugs such as high-dose aspirin and the corticosteroids. Table 26–1 is a review of the immunologic abnormalities and symptoms of each autoimmune disease reviewed in this chapter.

Suggested Readings

Stites, D. P., J. D. Stobo, H. H. Fudenberg and J. V. Wells. *Basic and Clinical Immunology*, 4th ed. Los Altos, CA: Lange Medical Publications, 1982.

Twomey, J. J., ed. *The Pathophysiology of Human Immunologic Disorders*. Baltimore, MD: Urban and Schwarzenberg, 1982.

REVIEW QUESTIONS for The Autoimmune Diseases

1. What is a common feature underlying all autoimmune diseases?

The common feature of all autoimmune diseases is that immunologic mechanisms (predominantly B- and T-lymphocyte clones) are activated which react against self molecules. [p. 157]

2. What abnormal anti-self immunoglobulin (ASI) is produced in the following autoimmune diseases?

Rheumatic fever	Anti-heart
Autoimmune thyroiditis	Anti-thyroid
Grave's Disease	Anti-thyroid gland receptor (LATS)
Goodpasture's syndrome	Anti-lung and kidney
Myasthenia gravis	Anti-neuromuscular junction
Autoimmune hemolytic anemia	Anti-red blood cell
Autoimmune thrombocytopenia	Anti-platelet
Autoimmune leukopenia	Anti-leukocyte
Aplastic anemia	Anti-stem cell
Systemic lupus erythematosus	Anti-nuclear
Rheumatoid arthritis	Anti-IgG (rheumatoid factor)

[p. 158]

Table 26–1. Immunologic Abnormalities and Symptoms of Some Representative Autoimmune Diseases.

Disease	***Abnormal Anti-Self Immunoglobulins (ASI) Produced***	***Symptoms***
Rheumatic fever	**Anti-heart**	**Heart inflammation**
Autoimmune thyroiditis	**Anti-thyroid**	**Hypothyroidism**
Grave's Disease	**Anti-thyroid gland receptor (LATS)**	**Hyperthyroidism**
Goodpasture's syndrome	**Anti-lung and kidney**	**Progressive lung and kidney failure**
Myasthenia gravis	**Anti-neuromuscular function**	**Progressive paralysis**
Autoimmune hemolytic anemia	**Anti-red blood cell**	**Anemia**
Autoimmune thrombocytopenia	**Anti-platelet**	**Bleeding**
Autoimmune leukopenia	**Anti-leukocyte**	**Infection**
Aplastic anemia	**Anti-stem cell**	**Decreased red blood cells, platelets, and leukocytes**
Systemic lupus erythematosis (SLE)	**Anti-nuclear**	**Immune-complex mediated inflammation of kidney, joints, skin, and central nervous system**
Rheumatoid arthritis	**Anti-IgG (rheumatoid factor)**	**Immune-complex mediated inflammation of joints and blood vessels**

3. What are the symptoms of the following autoimmune diseases?

Rheumatic fever	Heart inflammation
Autoimmune thyroiditis	Hypothyroidism
Grave's Disease	Hyperthyroidism
Goodpasture's syndrome	Progressive lung and kidney failure
Myasthenia gravis	Progressive paralysis
Autoimmune hemoloytic anemia	Anemia
Autoimmune thrombocytopenia	Bleeding
Autoimmune leukopenia	Infection
Aplastic anemia	Decreased red blood cells, platelets, and leukocytes
Systemic lupus erythematosus	Immune-complex mediated inflammation of kidney, joints, and skin
Rheumatoid arthritis	Immune complex-mediated inflammation of joints and blood vessels

[p. 158]

4. How are the following autoimmune diseases treated?

Rheumatic fever	Appropriate antibiotics are given to prevent anti-streptococcal idiotype from developing which cross-reacts with heart muscle. [p. 157]
Autoimmune thyroiditis	Thyroid hormone replacement. [p. 157]
Grave's disease	Specific drugs are given to block thyroid function, or thyroid cells can be eliminated by surgery or radiation therapy. [p. 157]
Goodpasture's syndrome	Plasmapheresis can remove circulating immunoglobulin, or poisonous toxins can be administered to kill the proliferating B-lymphocyte clones producing the autoimmune idiotype. [p. 158]
Myasthenia gravis	Treatment includes administration of various drugs that boost neuromuscular function (such as neostigmine), and plasmapheresis. [p. 158]
Autoimmune hemolytic anemia, autoimmune thrombocytopenia, autoimmune leukopenia, aplastic anemia	Treatment of these four disorders centers around removing the idiotype by reducing B-lymphocyte secretion of ASI by various drugs such as cyclophosphamide, or other treatments (such as splenectomy). [p. 158]
Systemic lupus erythematosus	Treatment includes the administration of certain drugs to inhibit B-lymphocyte secretion of ASI (such as cyclophosphamide). Corticosteroids and plasmapheresis are also employed. [p. 158]
Rheumatoid arthritis	Treatment centers around the use of various anti-inflammatory drugs (such as high-dose aspirin and corticosteroids). [p. 159]

CHAPTER 27

THE IMMUNODEFICIENCY DISEASES

Patients who suffer from immunodeficiency diseases all share a common defect in their immune system—the decreased ability to recognize and/or eliminate nonself invaders. As the old saying goes, "For every link in the chain, a break may occur." This adage seems applicable to the immunodeficiency diseases. By returning to Table 12–1 in Chapter 12 and Figure 21–1 in Chapter 21, the reader may review the four components of the immune system—the specific component of humoral immunity (immunoglobulin production), the nonspecific component of humoral immunity (complement), the specific component of cell-mediated immunity (T-lymphocyte function), and a nonspecific component of cell-mediated immunity (mononuclear phagocytes, PMN, and NK lymphocytes). In this chapter, each of these subcomponents is analyzed for defects as they relate to certain of the various immunodeficiency diseases currently known.

Immunodeficiency Diseases with Primary Defects in Antibody Production: Specific Humoral Immunity

There are four major disease groups that represent primary defects in immunoglobulin production: 1) decreased immunoglobulin production in infancy, called **hypogammaglobulinemia of infancy**; 2) **familial hypogammaglobulinemia**; 3) **common variable hypogammaglobulinemia**; and 4) **selective hypogammaglobulinemia**. *Hypogammaglobulinemia of infancy* is a self-limited disease that occurs in a small percentage of babies during the first six months of life. During the first six months, infants do not possess fully operational B lymphocytes for the production of normal levels of *IgG*; The IgG found in an infant's serum during this time is acquired from the mother prior to delivery. In hypogammaglobulinemia of infancy, for unknown reasons certain infants rapidly break down the IgG acquired from the mother. Thus, the infant is at an increased risk of infection during this period of time. Within six month's time the infant usually acquires normal antibody production without medical intervention.

Familial (congenital) hypogammaglobulinemia is the most clear cut example of severe impairment of immunoglobulin production. It involves *all* classes of immunoglobulin. The basic defect in this disease is an almost complete *absence of B lymphocytes* from the time of birth. The disease is transmitted genetically by a defect in one of the sex chromosomes; the disease usually appears in boys. The symptoms tend to appear very early in life, and the diagnosis is confirmed by demonstration of a near absence of B lymphocytes in the body, and consequently very low immunoglobulin levels in the serum. The most frequent complication of this disease is recurrent bacterial infection, but this can usually be controlled by the administration of purified immunoglobulins from normal donors.

Common variable hypogammaglobulinemia represents an acquired form of impaired immunoglobulin production which may occur at *any age* and in *either sex*. In most cases, common variable hypogammaglobulinemia represents a defect in the normal immunoregulatory mechanism for antibody production (see Figure 24–1 in Chapter 24) creating *nonfunctioning B lymphocytes*. The most frequently noted laboratory abnormality in this disease is the existence of an abnormally high number of *suppressor T lymphocytes* (that is, a decrease in the OKT4

/OKT8 ratio); the B- lymphocyte numbers are usually normal. Patients suffering from this disease may present with recurrent bacterial infections. Treatment currently centers around immunoglobulin replacement shots as needed. In the future it may be possible to administer biological response modifiers (BRM) to normalize the helper–suppressor (OKT4/OKT8) T-cell ratio, or to stimulate normal B- lymphocyte antibody production directly.

Selective hypogammaglobulinemia is usually an inherited defect in the ability of the patient to make only *one class* of antibody. The most frequent example of this disease is **selective IgA deficiency**. This disease is found in approximately 1 out of 600 individuals; it is usually **asymptomatic** (the patient may not show any visible symptoms) but it can be associated with recurrent upper respiratory infections and abdominal infections (because *IgA* protects those two areas from outside invasion). Treatment of the *symptoms* is usually the first line of therapy; replacement injections of immunoglobulin are sometimes indicated.

Immunodeficiency Disease Related to Defects in Complement Metabolism: Nonspecific Component of Humoral Immunity

There is a substantial list of immunodeficiency diseases that trace their origins to *defects in complement metabolism*. The best studied complement deficiency diseases are those that are inherited. They represent a genetically transmitted inability to synthesize certain of the complement components (Figure 19–1, Chapter 19). The most thoroughly studied diseases in this group are those demonstrating selective depressions in the amounts of the C5 through C8 complement components. In these diseases, the ability of patients to assemble the membrane attack complex ($\overline{C5,6,7,8,9}$) is impaired, and in laboratory measurements the blood levels of these specific components are found to be diminished. The blood levels show decreased serum C5 in selective C5 deficiency, decreased C6 in selective C6 deficiency, and so on. These patients may suffer from overwhelming bacterial infections, particularly a type of bacteria that causes gonorrhea or meningitis. Usually treatment for complement deficiency states is directed at treating any infections the patient might develop.

Immunodeficiency Diseases Reflecting Impaired T-Lymphocyte Function: Specific Cell-Mediated Immunity

The two best-studied diseases of T-lymphocyte function are the **DiGeorge syndrome** (present at birth) and the **acquired immunodeficiency syndrome (AIDS)**. The DiGeorge syndrome results from a defect during the maturation of the embryo which prevents the proper development of the *thymus gland*. Without a properly functioning thymus gland, the infant is unable to produce normally functioning *T-lymphocytes*. Patients with this disease suffer from recurrent tuberculosis and fungal and viral infections. Examination of their blood reveals a severe depression of T-lymphocyte numbers; B-lymphocyte numbers and immunoglobulin levels are normal. This disease is treated with thymus transplantation and with the infusion of biologic response modifiers (BRM) designed to augment T-lymphocyte function.

The acquired immunodeficiency syndrome (AIDS) is a newly recognized disease that is catastrophic in its effect and today is epidemic in its proportions. This disease afflicts previously normal individuals who most frequently belong to one of the following groups: 1) homosexuals and bisexuals, 2) abusers of injectable drugs, 3) hemophiliacs (or any patient receiving blood products), and 4) babies of infected mothers. The underlying cause of AIDS is thought to be a virus known as *human T-cell leukemia virus III (HTLV-III)*. The exact mechanism whereby the HTLV-III infection causes the AIDS syndrome is not understood, but the virus seems to prefer to infect helper T cells. This causes decreased release of helper T-lymphocyte lymphokines, thus paralyzing overall B- and T- lumphocyte and mononuclear phagocyte function (see Figure 27–1). Homosexual and bisexual males are the dominant group affected; the mode of trans-

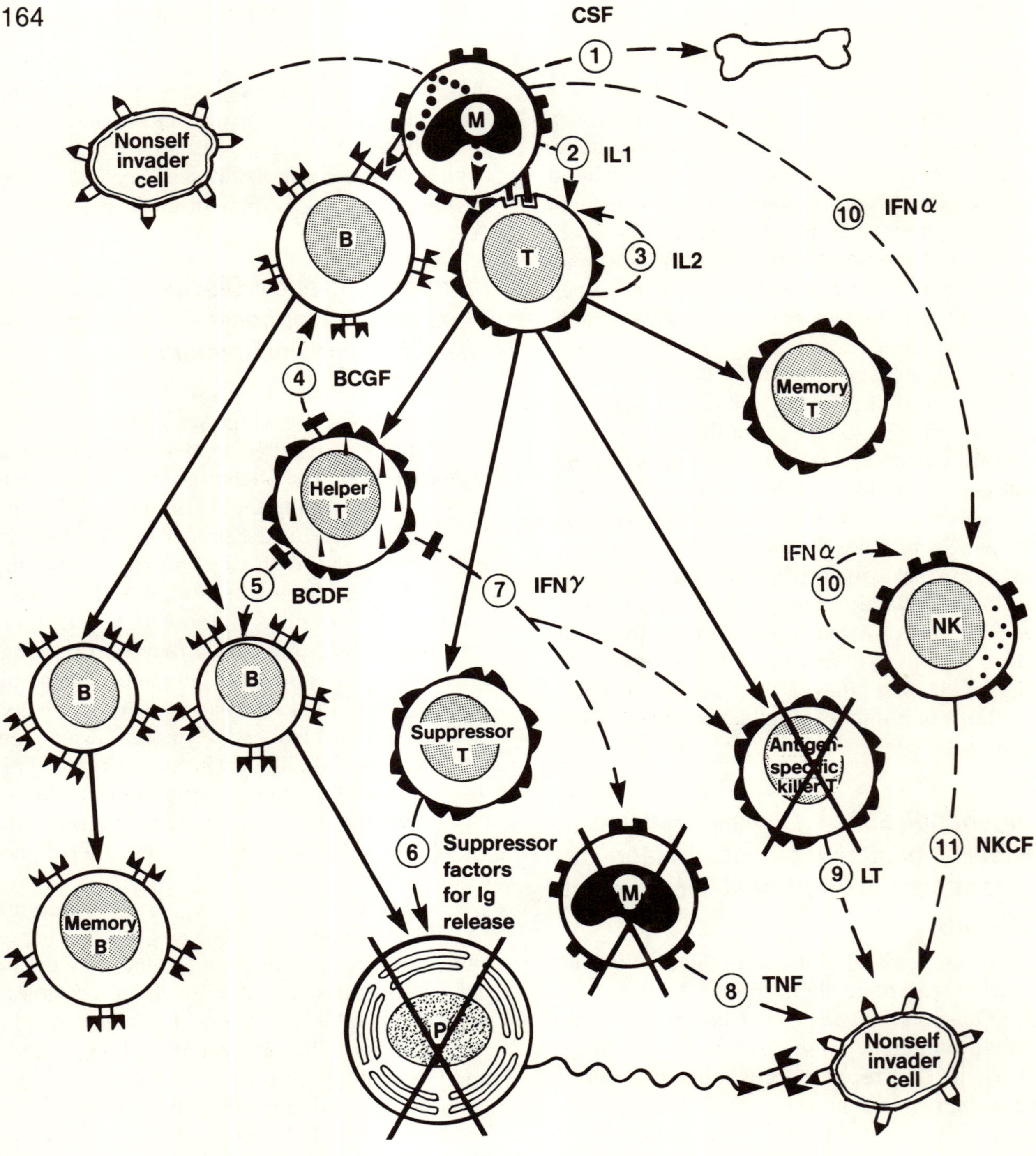

Key:						
B	=	B lymphocyte	LT	=	Lymphotoxin
BCDF	=	B-Cell Differentiation Factor	M	=	Mononuclear phagocyte
BCGF	=	B-Cell Growth Factor	NK	=	NK lymphocyte
CSF	=	Colony Stimulating Factor	NKCF	=	Natural Killer Cell Factor
IFN_γ	=	Interferon (gamma)	P	=	Plasma Cell
IFN_α	=	Interferon (alpha)	T	=	T lymphocyte
IL	=	Interleukin	TNF	=	Tumor Necrosis Factor
▲	=	HTLV-III virus			

Figure 27–1. Immunoregulation defects in patients with AIDS. HTLV-III virus (▲) infection of helper-T lymphocytes impairs B- and T-lymphocyte and mononuclear phagocyte function (⊗) and is related to deficient helper T-lymphocyte lymphokine release (– – █ – –).

mission appears to be through intimate sharing of body secretions. Casual social contact with these individuals does not appear to be a significant enough exposure to transmit the disease. Injectable drug abusers transmit the virus via contaminated needles. Hemophiliacs acquire the disease by receiving intravenous injections of blood products that were donated by AIDS patients. The disease is characterized by weight loss, enlargement of the lymph nodes, and recurrent tuberculosis, fungal, viral, and other opportunistic infections. These individuals also develop an increased susceptibility to the development of certain cancers such as **Kaposi's sarcoma**. Examination of patients' blood reveals lowered *helper T-lymphocyte* cell numbers (a decreased OKT4/OKT8 ratio). Treatment of the disease to date focuses on antibiotic therapy for the recurrent infections. Attempts are being made to treat these patients with biological response modifiers such as *gamma interferon* and *interleukin 2*, in an attempt to boost the failing T-lymphocyte system. Viral inhibitory drugs (such as **suramin** and **ribavirin**) are also being tested for this disease.

To prevent acquiring the disease, individuals should avoid intimate sexual contact with AIDS patients and should minimize the use of drug products that might be infected with the AIDS-causing virus (HTLV-III). A new blood screening test was recently developed that detects whether a prospective blood donor has been exposed to the AIDS virus. This test indicates that many people have been exposed to the HTLV-III virus but have not yet developed the full-blown AIDS disease. Some apparently normal individuals have evidence of the HTLV-III virus infection in their blood, but no symptoms. Others test positive to HTLV-III and present symptoms such as enlarged lymph nodes, fever, and weight loss (AIDS-related complex, ARC). These two groups of infected individuals are able to infect others and may develop the full-blown AIDS disease at a later time. Clearly, researchers must continue the attempt to develop a vaccine that will stimulate protective immunity against this deadly immunosuppressive virus.

Immunodeficiency Related to Defects in Mononuclear Phagocyte, PMN, and NK Lymphocyte Function: Nonspecific Component of Cell-Mediated Immunity

A few immunodeficiency diseases are thought to reflect a primary disturbance of the nonspecific component of cell-mediated immunity—the *mononuclear phagocytes*, *PMN*, and *NK lymphocytes*. Two well-studied diseases representing defects in the nonspecific component of cellular immunity are the **Chediak-Higashi syndrome** and **chronic granulomatous disease (CGD)**. These diseases represent two distinct defects in the cellular mechanisms required to kill infectious agents once they are ingested by mononuclear phagocytes and PMN. For this reason, both Chediak-Higashi syndrome patients and patients with CGD are very susceptible to serious recurrent infections. There is some evidence that the NK lymphocyte function of these patients is also abnormal. Patients with these diseases who survive into their twenties frequently develop cancer. Treatment of both diseases at this time is mainly supportive; antibiotics are given to treat infections as they develop.

Perhaps the most common immune deficiency relative to mononuclear phagocytes, PMN, and NK lymphocytes is seen in cancer patients treated with chemotherapeutic agents. These anti-cancer cell poisons also kill some normal cells, including the stem cell that gives rise to these nonspecific cell-mediated immune system cells. During chemotherapy treatments, the numbers of circulating PMN, monocytes, and NK lymphocytes diminishes in the blood. Chemotherapy is a period in which cancer patients are at very high risk of infection. The treatment for this drug-induced disease involves supporting the patient with antibiotics until the effects of the chemotherapy wear off and the numbers of mononuclear phagocytes, PMN, and NK lymphocytes return to normal.

Combined Immunodeficiency Diseases

A number of diseases appear to be **mixed immune deficiencies**. They involve defects both in humoral and cell-mediated immunity. These diseases are known collectively as **severe combined immunodeficiency (SCID) syndromes**. These syndromes are all hereditary diseases that usually present in infancy as overwhelming bacterial, viral, and fungal infections. Examination of the white cells of these patients reveals that both *T- and B-lymphocyte* numbers usually are markedly diminished, and serum *immunoglobulin* levels may be quite low. These very severe immunodeficiency diseases reflect a defect at the level of a common differentiation factor required for normal T- and B-lymphocyte function. In addition to receiving antibiotic support when needed, these patients are treated with bone marrow transplantation and with biological response modifier infusion designed to boost both humoral and cell-mediated immunity. Refer to Table 27–1 for a listing of these diseases and their characteristics.

Suggested Reading

Barrett, J. T. *Textbook of Immunology*. St. Louis, MO: Mosby, 1983.

Hood, L. E., I. L. Weissman, W. B. Wood, and J. H. Wilson. *Immunology*. Menlo Park, CA: Benjamin/Cummings, 1984.

Table 27–1. Characteristics of the Immunodeficiency Diseases.

Disease	Immune System Subcomponent Affected	Symptoms
Hypogammaglobulinemia of infancy	B lymphocyte	Recurrent bacterial infections for first 6 months of life
Familial hypogammablobulinemia	B lymphocyte	Lifelong recurrent bacterial infections
Common variable hypogammaglobulinemia	B lymphocyte	Acquired predisposition to bacterial infections
Selective hypogammaglobulinemia	B lymphocyte	Hereditary IgA deficiency—usually asymptomatic
C5 through C8 deficiency	Complement	Lifelong predisposition to gonorrhea or meningitis
DiGeorge syndrome	T lymphocyte	Lifelong recurrent tuberculosis, fungal and viral infections
Acquired immunodeficiency syndrome (AIDS)	T lymphocyte	Acquired predisposition to opportunistic infections; Kaposi's sarcoma
Chediak-Higashi syndrome and chronic granulomatous disease (CGD)	Mononuclear phagocytes, PMN and NK lymphocytes	Lifelong predisposition to bacterial and fungal infections
Severe combined immunodeficiency (SCID)	B and T lymphocytes	Lifelong recurrent bacterial, fungal, and viral infections

REVIEW QUESTIONS for The Immunodeficiency Diseases

1. What do all immunodeficiency diseases share in common?

All demonstrate a compromised ability to recognize and/or eliminate nonself invaders. [p. 162]

2. Name four major disease groups that represent primary defects in immunoglobulin production.

1) Hypogammaglobulinemia of infancy
2) Familial hypogammaglobulinemia
3) Common variable hypogammaglobulinemia
4) Selective hypogammaglobulinemia

[p. 162]

3. What is the cause of the acquired immunodeficiency syndrome (AIDS)?

The HTLV-III virus (which infects helper T lymphocytes) causes AIDS. [p. 163]

4. What immune system subcomponent is affected in the following immunodeficiency diseases?

Hypogammaglobulinemia of infancy?	B lymphocyte
Familial hypogammaglobulinemia	B lymphocyte
Common variable hypogammaglobulinemia	B lymphocyte
Selective hypogammaglobulinemia	B lymphocyte
C5 through C8 deficiency	Complement
DiGeorge syndrome	T lymphocyte
Acquired immunodeficiency syndrome (AIDS)	Helper T lymphocytes
Chediak-Higashi syndrome and chronic granulomatous disease (CGD)	Mononuclear phagocytes, PMN, and NK lymphocytes
Combined immunodeficiency	B and T lymphocytes

[p. 166]

5. What symptoms are related to the following immunodeficiency diseases?

Hypogammaglobulinemia of infancy	Recurrent bacterial infections for the first 6 months of life
Familial hypogammaglobulinemia?	Lifelong recurrent bacterial infections
Common variable hypogammaglobulinemia	Acquired predisposition to bacterial infections
Selective hypogammaglobulinemia	IgA deficiency is usually asymptomatic.
C5 through C8 deficiency	Lifelong predisposition to gonorrhea or meningitis
DiGeorge syndrome	Lifelong recurrent tuberculosis, fungal and viral infections
Acquired immunodeficiency syndrome (AIDS)	Acquired predisposition to opportunistic infections plus cancers, such as Kaposi's sarcoma
Chediak-Higashi syndrome and CGD	Lifelong predisposition to bacterial and fungal infections

Combined immunodeficiency	Lifelong recurrent bacterial, fungal, and viral infections [p. 166]
6. What is the AIDS-related complex (ARC)?	ARC is the fever, weight loss, and lymph node enlargement in individuals who have evidence of exposure to the HTLV-III virus (they do not have the full-blown AIDS syndrome, however). [p. 165]
7. What is the current treatment for the following immunodeficiency diseases?	
Hypogammaglobulinemia of infancy	Immunoglobulin replacement if needed during the first 6 months of life
Familial hypogammaglobulinemia	Lifelong immunoglobulin replacement
Common variable hypogammaglobulinemia	Immunoglobulin replacement as needed
C5 through C8 deficiency	Antibiotic therapy for infections
DiGeorge syndrome	Thymus replacement and BRM therapy
AIDS	Antibiotic therapy and antiviral drug therapy (such as suramin and ribavirin) and BRM administration (such as IFN_{γ} and IL2)
Chediak-Higashi syndrome and CGD	Antibiotic therapy as needed
Combined immunodeficiency	Antibiotic therapy, BRM administration, and bone marrow transplantation [p. 165]

CHAPTER 28

TRANSPLANTATION AND IMMUNOTHERAPY

A new discipline in medicine emerged since the 1970s, namely the replacement of diseased human organs with healthy organs obtained from volunteers or cadavers. The field of **transplantation medicine** includes the transplantation of kidneys, hearts, bone marrow, and other organs. The surgical component of transplantation medicine is relatively straightforward: the surgeon needs to connect the blood supply of the transplanted organ to the blood vessels of the patient. The major problem in transplantation medicine centers around the patient's immunologic reaction to the nonself invasion of the body by the transplanted tissue.

The critical element is *how long* a transplanted organ will survive in a patient's body. This is determined by how well the *HLA type* of the organ donor correlates with the HLA type of the cells of the patient. In an organ transplantation between HLA-matched identical twins, for example, the organ has a 100 percent chance of survival at the end of 5 years. However, if the HLA type of the transplanted organ is mismatched to the HLA type of the patient, even with the most aggressive therapy there is less than a 50 percent chance that the organ will remain functioning at the end of 5 years. The closer the HLA type of the transplanted organ is to the HLA type of the patient, the greater the chance of survival of the graft.

In addition to sensitive tests that allow physicians to match the HLA type of the organ to the HLA type of the patient as much as possible, two other advances have contributed to the survival of transplant patients. First, there are substantial advances in the recognition of the mechanism of graft rejection and how to treat it. One component of **graft rejection** involves the formation of *antibodies* against antigens found on the transplanted organ. If allowed to progress, this *humoral immune response* against the transplanted organ will cause failure of the transplanted organ within a week. More commonly, transplant patients frequently develop *cell-mediated immunity* against the transplanted organ with actual infiltration of the organ by antigen-specific *T lymphocytes* and recruited nonspecific effector cells (PMN, NK cells, and mononuclear phagocytes). For this reason, most transplant patients are treated with high doses of drugs that dampen the immune response, called **immunosuppressive agents**. These include corticosteroids, chemotherapeutic agents such as cyclophosphamide and azothiaprine, and, most recently, an agent known as cyclosporin A. Patients tend to require these immunosuppressive regimens for a long period of time, until their physicians are certain that the risk of organ transplantation has passed.

The second advance in transplantation medicine is an improvement in physicians' ability to support transplant patients during the risk period of frequent complications. Perhaps the most common problem is *repeated infections* due to the immunosuppression created by the immunosuppressive drugs. Transplantation medical teams now know how to diagnose and treat infections as early as possible, supporting the patient through this critical period.

Another transplantation reaction is that of **blood transfusion reactions**. Patients with low red blood cell counts (*anemia*) require treatment with intravenous infusions of red blood cells obtained from healthy individuals as needed.

Red blood cell transfusions following accidental or surgical blood loss can save lives; certain patients (such as those suffering from *aplastic anemia*—see Chapter 26) require blood transfusions on a regular basis. In all cases it is very important to match as closely as possible the red blood cell type of the blood donor to the red blood cell type of the recipient.

There are many distinct blood group antigens on human red blood cells, and they vary in clinical importance. The immunologic concepts pertinent to the principal blood group, the ABO system, are presented here; these general principles are applicable to other blood group antigens as well. Human red blood cells have two major antigens on their surfaces; one is sugar called **A**, and the other is a different sugar known as **B**. These two blood group antigens are the products of two enzymes that derive in turn from two distinct alleles occupying the *major blood cell antigen gene site* (the ABO locus). Thus, of the two matching genes that code for the major red blood cell antigens, an individual can inherit two A alleles, two B alleles, or an A allele and a B allele. There is a third, *nonfunctional*, allele known as the **O** allele. It is perhaps easy to think of the name of this allele as the *zero* allele because it does not code for any functional enzyme protein (thus, no sugar is produced). The red blood cells of an individual who inherits two O alleles will not express either the A or the B sugars, and the red blood cell type of that individual will be O. The red blood cells of an individual who inherits an A allele and an O allele will express only A sugars, and thus that person will have blood group type A. Likewise, the red blood cells of an individual who inherits a B allele and an O allele will express only B sugars and will be said to have a B red blood cell type. Thus, there are two ways an individual can inherit an A red blood cell phenotype: by having two A alleles or by having an A allele and an O allele genotype. There are also two ways to inherit a B red blood cell phenotype: by inheriting two B alleles or by inheriting a B allele and an O allele genotype. There is only one way an individual can have an AB red blood cell phenotype: by inheriting one A and one B allele genotype. Finally, there is only one way an individual can inherit an O red blood cell phenotype: by inheriting *two* O alleles as the genotype.

There is another fact to remember in order to understand red blood cell transfusion reactions. Individuals of a specific blood type have naturally occurring antibodies in their blood which are reactive to blood groups *other than the one possessed by that person*. That is to say, the bloodstream of an individual with type A red blood cells has anti-B immunoglobulin. Likewise, the bloodstream of an individual with type B red blood cells has naturally occurring anti-A immunoglobulin. In contrast, the bloodstream of an individual with type O red blood cells has both anti-A and anti-B immunoglobulin. Because an individual with the AB red blood cell type has *both* antigens, no immunoglobulin against red blood cells will be found in the serum of this individual. The mechanism for production of immunoglobulin reactive to other red blood cell types (in patients who have never been previously transfused) is thought to happen when individuals are infected with bacteria that have surface antigens similar to red blood cell group types. Thus, in the process of making antibodies against certain bacteria, these patients also create anti-red blood cell antibodies that react with red blood cells of a type different from their own. Obviously, it would be very harmful if an individual made an antibody that cross-reacted between bacterial antigens and his or her own red blood cells because this would cause autoimmune hemolytic anemia (Chapter 26).

As shown in Figure 28–1, once you understand the A, B, and O red blood cell antigen system and you remember the fact that individuals will naturally make immunoglobulin (antibodies) against the red blood cell antigens that they do not possess, it is easy to predict red blood cell transfusion reactions. **Transfusion reactions** are characterized by the acute onset of fever and malaise when incompatible blood is given to a patient. The patient's kidneys may be damaged by the release of too much hemoglobin from the transfused red blood cells that are damaged by the antibodies found in the patient's bloodstream. Individuals with the red blood cell type O have both anti-A and anti-B

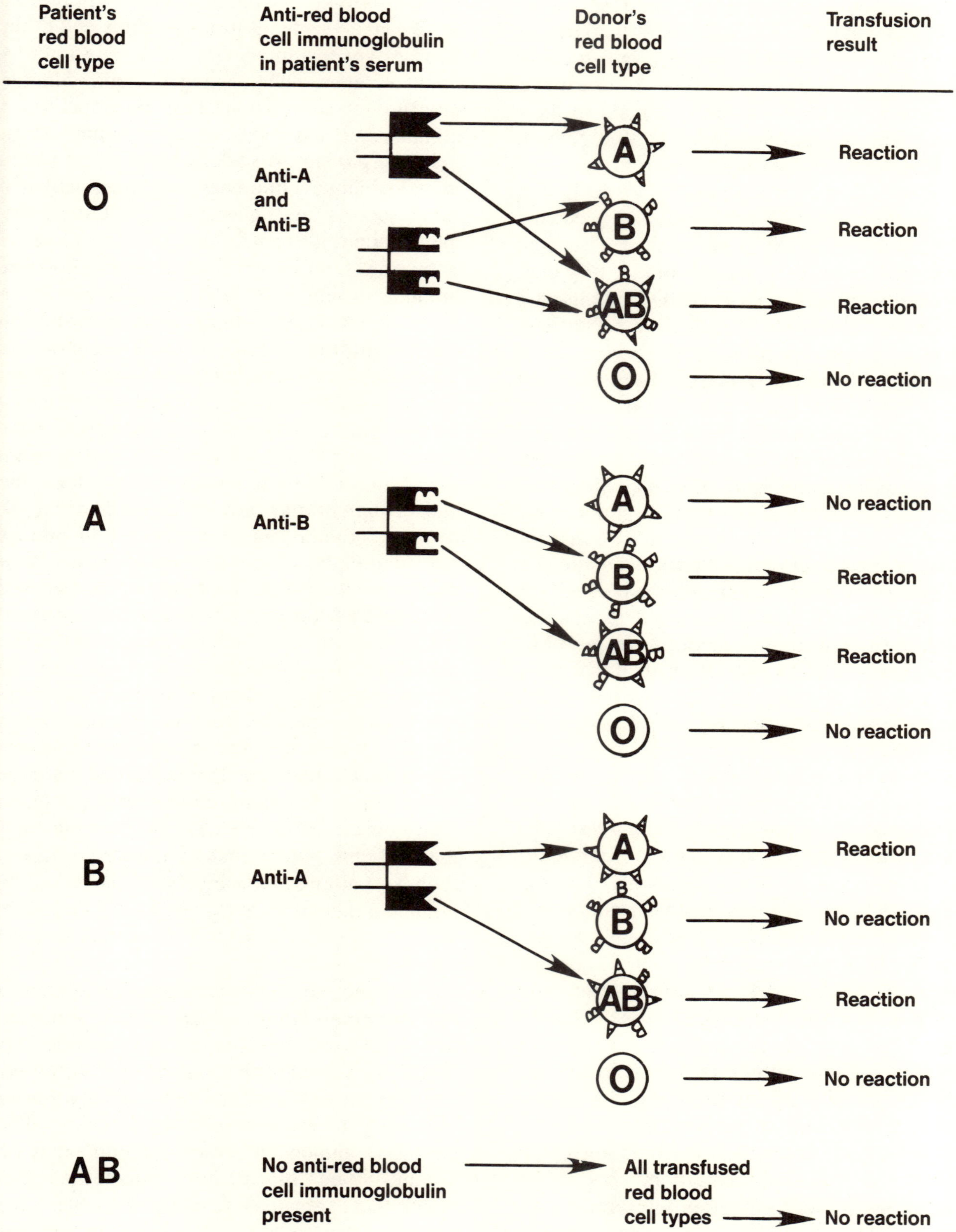

Figure 28–1. Mechanism for red blood cell transfusion reactions.

immunoglobulin in their serum and react to the red blood cell types A, B, and AB; the only red blood cell type that they can receive is type O. Individuals with blood cell type A have naturally occurring anti-B immunoglobulin in their serum. They cannot receive red blood cells of the B or AB type; they can, however, receive A and O red blood cells. Likewise, individuals with type B red blood cells have naturally occurring anti-A immunoglobulin in their serum. They cannot receive type A or type AB blood; they can, however, receive type B or type O. Patients who have type AB red blood cells have no anti-red blood cell immunoglobulins in their serum. Thus, these individuals can receive all types of red blood cells (but not whole blood). For this reason, the patient with the AB red blood cell type is frequently called the **universal recipient**. As you can see from Figure 28–1, all patients can receive type O blood; so type O patients are frequently called **universal donors**. The therapy for transfusion reactions centers around attempting to prevent kidney damage by the hemoglobin released from the damaged red blood cells. Because most transfusion reactions are preventable with adequate laboratory evaluations, every effort should be made to ensure red blood cell compatibility prior to the initiation of any transfusion.

For several hundred years, attempts have been made to decrease the susceptibility of humans to all forms of nonself invasion. **Natural resistance** refers to the inherited (not acquired) immunity of an individual. **Acquired immunity** develops after birth following exposure to certain nonself invaders. For many decades physicians have successfully boosted acquired immunity to certain infectious diseases by the administration of nonlethal forms of the infectious agent. In the United States today, for example, children are immunized against diptheria, pertussis, and tetanus (**DPT**) with injections containing tetanus and diptheria toxoids (modified bacterial toxins) and killed pertussis bacteria; these injections are given at 2, 4, 6, 18, and 48 months of age. An oral polio vaccine is given following a similar schedule. A vaccine of nonvirulent measles virus and mumps virus is given at 15 months of age. In adulthood it is recommended that tetanus toxoid booster injections be given every 10 to 12 years; vaccinations to smallpox and other diseases are recommended for certain international travelers. The boosting of acquired immunity through stimulation of an individual's own immune system is known as **active immunization**.

In the past few decades another type of immunologic intervention has been attempted with some success in cancer patients. **Cancer immunotherapy** is the treatment of the patient's immune system in a way that might allow the immune system cells of the cancer patient to fight off and possibly eliminate the nonself invasion of the tumor cells. A current hypothesis holds that the major defect in the cancer patient may not necessarily be the presence of tumor cells but rather a weakness in the patient's immune system which prevents the patient from destroying his or her tumor cell burden. The cancer patient may have a decreased ability to *recognize* tumor cells as nonself, and/or may have decreased ability to *destroy* these tumor cells once recognized. Because it is believed that the development of cancer cells (nonself transformation) may occur normally and as frequently as on a daily basis, it is felt that the immune system may help to identify and eliminate newly emerging tumor cells day-to-day. Thus, if there is a defect in the immune system function, it follows that a patient might be prone to develop a malignant (cancerous) disease. In fact, some clinical evidence to date indicates that patients with impaired immune systems, such as patients suffering from the acquired immunodeficiency syndrome (AIDS), have substantially increased risks of developing certain cancers.

Two major strategies are currently employed in the *immunotherapy of cancer*. One approach is to adminster biological response modifiers (BRM) to stimulate the immune system of the cancer patient to function perhaps more efficiently in the destruction of tumor cells. Currently, biological response modifiers, such as the alpha and gamma interferons and interleukin 2, are given to cancer patients to see if the immune system function of these patients is improved and if the established tumor can be eliminated. It is clear that to date no *one* biological response modifier is effective as a treatment for all types of cancer. However, several exciting regressions of certain types of malignancies occur when specific biological response modifiers are administered. One example is a form of leukemia known as **hairy-cell leukemia**. When patients are exposed to **alpha interferon** by intramuscular injection, a striking regression of all observable tumor is noted in most of the patients treated to date. The exact mechanism for the regression of cancer in patients receiving this and similar types of biological response modifier therapy is not known. One possibility, however, is that these agents boost the immune system function as shown in Figure 28–2.

Another promising form of biological response modifier therapy is administration of tumor-specific *monoclonal antibodies* to cancer patients. It is known that these antibodies, once they are injected, will "home" to the tumor cells. It is hoped that monoclonal antibodies bound to tumor cells might then focus nonspecific immune functions (complement and/or ADCC effector cells) to eliminate the tumor cells. Because antibodies from outside the host are added, this is a form of **passive immunity** (as compared to *active immunity*, described previously. However, to date, no specific activation of the complement cascade, or of the nonspecific cell-mediated immune system component, has been noted in the area of monoclonal antibody-coated tumor cells. It is felt that perhaps monoclonal antibodies derived from mice may not be capable of activating these two nonself invader clearance systems. In addition, because murine (mouse-derived) monoclonal antibodies are considered foreign to humans, several hypersensitivity reactions have been observed in some patients treated to date. Nevertheless, tumor-specific monoclonal antibodies tagged with toxins or radioactive substances may be used to concentrate these cellular poisons on the tumor cells in the cancer patient's body. Clinical experimentation with this approach is currently under way.

Immunotherapeutic strategy, also recently tested in cancer patients, is removal of various anti-tumor leukocytes from the cancer patient's body. The leukocytes are activated to **tumoricidal** (tumor killing) **activity** in the test tube (*in vitro*),

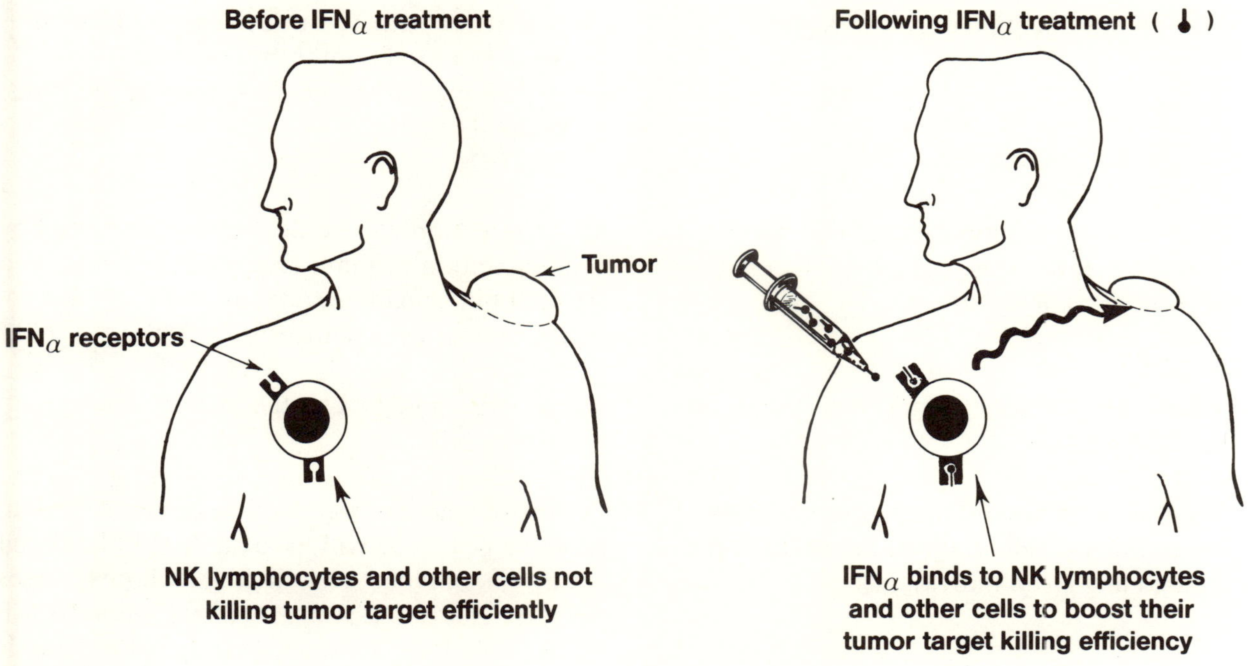

Figure 28–2. Possible mechanism of action of alpha interferon (IFN$_\alpha$) in the treatment of cancer patients.

and then reinfused directly to the sites of tumor in the patient. Two cell types are currently being evaluated in this regard, as summarized in Figure 28–3. In one study, *lymphocytes* are removed from the patient's body, activated with a lymphokine (*interleukin 2*), and reinfused back into the patient along with additional IL2. These *lymphokine-activated killer lymphocytes (or LAK cells)* are quite tumoricidal when exposed to cancer cells *in vitro*. It is hoped that they may be active in the cancer patient as well. Similarly, blood *monocytes* are removed from cancer patients, activated with *gamma interferon* to tumoricidal activity *in vitro*, and then reinfused to the site of the patient's tumor along with additional IFN_a. This clinical project is termed the **ex-vivo leukocyte activation (or EVLA) protocol** (or therapy). Because monocytes display potent anti-tumor functions in the test tube, it is hoped that clinical results in cancer patients may be equally promising.

Suggested Reading

Hood, L. E., I. L. Weissman, W. B. Wood, and J. H. Wilson. *Immunology*. Menlo Park, CA: Benjamin/Cummings, 1984.

Stites, D. P., J. B. Stobo, H. H. Fudenberg, and J. B. Wells. *Basic and Clinical Immunology*, 4th ed. Los Altos, CA: Lange Medical Publications, 1982.

REVIEW QUESTIONS for Transplantation and Tumor Immunology

1. What is the most important predictor of the success of organ transplantation?

   Organ transplantation requires successful matching of the transplanted organ's HLA type with the patient's HLA type. (An ABO system match is also desirable.) [p. 169]

2. What are the two mechanisms by which a patient can reject an organ transplant?

   1) Rejection by the production of antibodies that react with the transplanted organ antigens (humoral immunity); or
   2) by cell-mediated immunity against the transplanted organ.
   [p. 169]

3. How can the humoral and cell-mediated graft rejection of a transplanted organ be prevented or delayed?

   Graft rejection can be delayed or prevented by administration of immunosuppressive drugs such as cyclophosphamide, azothiaprine, corticosteroids, and/or cyclosporin A. [p. 169]

4. What are the four major red blood cell group types?

   A, B, AB, and O are the major RBC group types. [p. 170]

5. What are the six different combinations of the red blood cell group alleles that are possible in any given individual?

   A person who has two A alleles or an A and an O allele genotype will have an A red blood cell group phenotype. An individual who expresses two B alleles or a B and an O allele genotype will have a type B red blood cell group phenotype. If the individual has an A allele and a B allele genotype, the AB red blood cell group pheno-

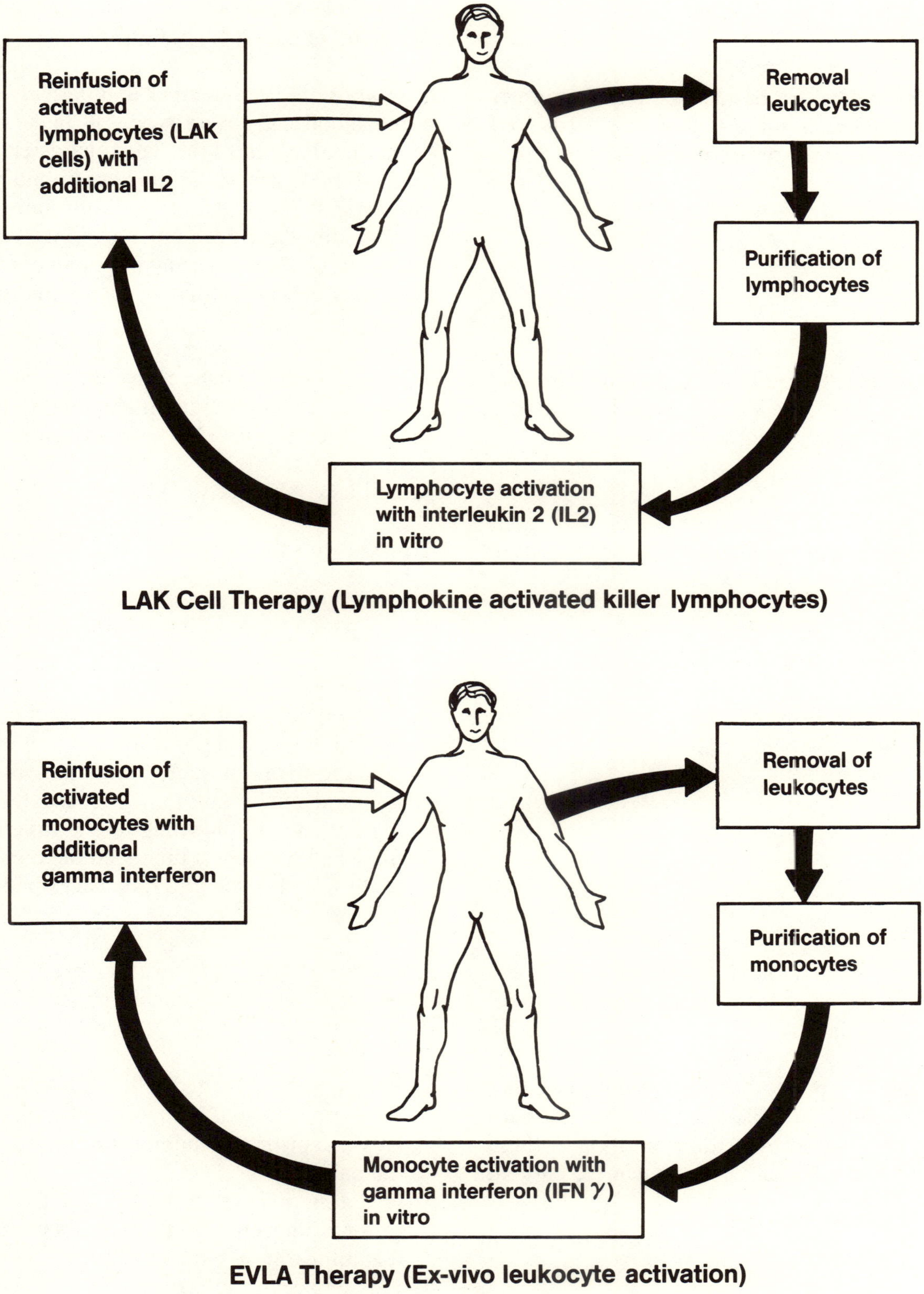

Figure 28–3. Two forms of adoptive cellular immunotherapy for cancer.

type will be expressed. An individual who has two O allele genotypes will have an O red blood cell group phenotype. [p. 170]

6. What other fact besides the blood group of the patient is important in predicting red blood cell transfusion reactions?

It is important to remember that patients of the A red blood cell group type will make anti-B antibodies. Patients of the B red blood cell group type will make anti-A antibodies. An individual with type O blood will make both anti-A and anti-B antibodies; however, an individual with AB blood will not have any naturally occurring red blood cell antibodies in his or her serum. [p. 170]

7. What type of red blood cells can be infused into a type A patient, a type B patient, a type O patient, and a type AB patient?

The type A patient can receive type A and type O blood. The type B patient can receive type B and type O blood. The type AB patient can receive A, B, AB, or O blood. The type O patient can only receive O blood. [p. 171]

8. What type of red blood cell donor is considered the universal donor?

Type O is the universal donor. [p. 172]

9. What type of red blood cell donor is considered the universal recipient?

Type AB is the universal recipient. [p. 172]

10. What two forms of cancer immunotherapy are currently being employed?

1) Administration of biological response modifiers to the patient in an attempt to boost the immune system function of the patient.
2) Removal of the anti-tumor leukocytes from the patient, the boosting of the function of these cells in the test tube, and the reinfusion of these cells back into the cancer patient.

[p. 172]

11. Name some biological response modifiers that have been used in cancer patient treatment to date.

Alpha interferon, gamma interferon, and interleukin 2 are given to cancer patients. [p. 173]

12. Name two protocols that attempt to remove the anti-tumor leukocytes from the patient's body, followed by readministration of these activated cells back into the cancer patient.

1) Lymphokine-activated killer (LAK) lymphocytes are activated in the test tube with interleukin 2 prior to readministration back into the patient.
2) Blood monocytes have been activated by gamma interferon in the test tube prior to readministration back into patients in the *ex-vivo* leukocyte activation (EVLA) research project.

[p. 174]

INDEX

*Boldface type indicates page where term is defined.